BEYOND KETO

DON COLBERT, MD

SILOAM

Most Charisma Media products are available at special quantity discounts for bulk purchase for sales promotions, premiums, fund-raising, and educational needs. For details, call us at (407) 333-0600 or visit our website at www.charismamedia.com.

Beyond Keto by Don Colbert, MD
Published by Siloam, an imprint of Charisma Media
600 Rinehart Road, Lake Mary, Florida 32746

Visit the author's website at drcolbert.com, www.drcolbertbooks.com.

Cataloging-in-Publication Data is on file with the Library of Congress.
International Standard Book Number: 978-1-63641-070-8
E-book ISBN: 978-1-63641-071-5

This book contains the opinions and ideas of its author. It is solely for informational and educational purposes and should not be regarded as a substitute for professional medical treatment. The nature of your body's health condition is complex and unique. Therefore, you should consult a health professional before you begin any new exercise, nutrition, or supplementation program or if you have questions about your health. Neither the author nor the publisher shall be liable or responsible for any loss or damage allegedly arising from any information or suggestion in this book.

People and names in this book are composites created by the author from his experiences as a medical doctor. Names and details of their stories have been changed, and any similarity between the names and stories of individuals described in this book and individuals known to readers is purely coincidental.

22 23 24 25 26 — 9 8 7 6 5 4 3 2 1
Printed in the United States of America

This book is dedicated to my patients, who are committed to walking in divine health. Finally there is a lifestyle program that will enable them to live a long and healthy life generally resistant to disease. You catch a cold or the flu, but you develop disease by consistently making the wrong food and beverage choices. Beyond Keto provides a road map for choosing healthy foods and beverages to lose weight, prevent most diseases, and for many, even reverse disease. My patients have fueled my desire to research and find the answers to their health problems. I have found that there is no magic supplement, vitamin, or medicine that will cure most diseases. The best solution is simply letting your food be your medicine. Beyond Keto is a tool for doing just that. To your health!

CONTENTS

PART I: THE INS AND OUTS OF KETO

PART II: THE MEDITERRANEAN-KETO LIFESTYLE

PART III: RECIPES FOR A HEALTHY MEDITERRANEAN-KETO LIFESTYLE

ACKNOWLEDGMENTS

I WANT TO GIVE special thanks to Efie Gialedakis, our dear friend from Crete, Greece. She traveled with us throughout Crete and Athens and introduced us to high-polyphenol olive oil that is high in oleocanthal, one of the most powerful phytonutrients in the world. She also introduced me to Prokopios Magiatis, PhD, at the University of Athens, who is a world authority on olive oil and especially oleocanthal. I am grateful to Dr. Magiatis for letting me spend more than three hours with him at the university during my trip.

PREFACE

N OT LONG AGO I visited an island in Greece where people have grown olives and produced olive oil for thousands of years. The island actually has an olive tree that is over two thousand years old!

While enjoying their Mediterranean cuisine and slower-paced lifestyle, I had an epiphany. These people live longer than almost everyone else on the planet. They have answers that we on a Western diet with our ever-expanding waistlines and list of sicknesses and diseases should really stop and learn.

I understood the power of the Mediterranean diet, and it didn't take me long to see that here was an entire group of people living the Mediterranean lifestyle. They ate that way at home. They ate that way in restaurants. And they have been eating that way for centuries.

Yet they smoke! At 39.1 percent, Greece, of all the countries in the world, has the ninth-highest percentage of people aged fifteen and older who smoke.[1] In the United States roughly 14 percent of adults smoke cigarettes.[2] Yet Greece has lower numbers for heart disease and cancer, as well as obesity.[3]

The answers are always in the food. Here was a living, breathing Mediterranean lifestyle right in front of me—and it worked. What's more, they had years and years of research and results on the medical side of things as undeniable proof.

That is where we are going with this book. We start with a healthy keto diet (part 1) and work out all the kinks that have tripped up many people on a typical keto diet. Then we move over into a Mediterranean-keto lifestyle (part 2).

It's the same diet, just tweaked and adjusted a bit so you can live in the sweet spot that prevents most sicknesses and diseases while simultaneously bringing you incredible health and vitality.

That's where we are going. I welcome you to join me.

—DON COLBERT, MD

INTRODUCTION

O NE EPIDEMIC RESPONSIBLE for countless diseases, sicknesses, and unfulfilled lives is the obesity epidemic, and it is only getting worse. I wrote *Dr. Colbert's Keto Zone Diet* in 2017 to help combat that epidemic. After all, obesity is the root cause of most of the diseases we face today. Thousands of readers were able to lose weight and control their appetites. The keto diet worked wonders!

As a practicing physician, I continued to work with patients and kept looking for ways to improve their lives. That's what I've done and will always do.

Unexpectedly, I began to hear that many people on the keto diet, including some of my patients, were being placed on statin medications to lower their cholesterol. For many, their cholesterol had gone up fifty to one hundred points!

This didn't make sense, because lower cholesterol is usually a natural result of a healthy keto diet. And higher cholesterol was not the only problem. Some keto diet followers were developing other issues as well, such as

- joint pain

- muscle aches

- nasal congestion

- sinus issues

- fatigue

- brain fog

- memory problems

- gut issues (constipation; irritable bowel syndrome, or IBS; food allergies; food sensitivities; etc.)

- prediabetes
- type 2 diabetes
- heart disease
- hypertension
- cancer
- weight gain (on occasion).

Statin medication for high cholesterol can actually cause some of these very symptoms, but these symptoms were being experienced by many keto dieters before they went to their primary physician and were placed on statin drugs. Obviously something in the keto diet was not working.

So I dug a little deeper. I read, researched, studied, compared, and prodded my patients with questions. As a result, I found several gaping holes that apply to virtually everyone on the keto diet.

We will discuss these holes in the typical keto diet in the pages to come, but the most common and biggest hole affects 80 percent of keto dieters. It's more than a hole, really; it's more like a sinkhole that swallowed the entire road!

Let me explain. People like the keto diet and the benefits that come with it, but on average only about 20 percent of people or less actually stay with it long term. That's the norm with any diet.[1] Only a few will stick with it, and usually it's those with a motivation (disease, health, lifestyle, etc.) so strong that they keep going no matter what. When it's doctor's orders in a life-or-death situation, they really stick with it, but not everyone is in such a tough situation when they choose the keto diet.

The remaining 80 percent keep what they had come to enjoy on the keto diet—such as butter, cream, cheese, coconut oil, and fatty meats that they ate while losing weight—as they go back to their normal American diets with excessive sugars, carbs, and starches.

It may seem like a minor issue, but that is the number one problem. The vast majority of keto dieters combine their new and old eating habits together. They mix the eating of a lot of saturated fats with the usual high-carb, starchy, sugary American diet.

The direct result: inflammation! No wonder their bad cholesterol levels were going up. Inflammation is a root cause of almost all chronic diseases, including cardiovascular disease, arthritis, most cancers, autoimmune diseases, even Alzheimer's disease and Parkinson's disease. It turns out that saturated fats cause inflammation, especially when eaten with refined carbohydrates or sugars or when you don't have enough omega-3 fats (fish oil) in your body.[2]

On the keto diet, with sufficient omega-3 and the very low carbs, starches, and sugar, keto dieters were, for the most part, able to get away with eating a lot of saturated fats. But once they went back to their normal American diet, the mixing of saturated fats with carbs and sugar caused inflammation, not to mention weight gain.

But that was not all. The high amount of saturated fats was also causing insulin resistance, which has been found to be a root cause of prediabetes, type 2 diabetes, Alzheimer's, Parkinson's, and many more of the more than one hundred autoimmune diseases.

Something had to change, and quickly! The keto diet is good, and it is still the absolute best way to lose weight, maintain a healthy metabolism, and fight sickness and disease (even cancers), but if the vast majority of people eventually revert back to their old eating habits, then the healthy benefits of a keto diet will begin to unravel.

I knew there had to be a better way. There had to be an option that provided the benefits of a keto diet with a lifestyle that could be lived and enjoyed long term. And there is an answer! Reduced to two simple steps, here is the answer:

> Step 1: Start with a healthy keto diet to lose weight, gain health benefits, or treat or prevent sickness or disease. That is part 1 of this book.

> Step 2: Then slide over to a healthy Mediterranean-keto lifestyle that enables you to keep the weight off, be healthy, and avoid sickness and disease. That is part 2 of this book.

The answer, where all this is taking us, is a lifestyle that mixes the benefits of a keto diet with the joy and practicality of a healthy lifestyle. To prove my point, you can jump right into the Mediterranean-keto lifestyle if you want, and you will still lose weight (just more slowly) and still get all the health benefits of the keto diet.

As for rising cholesterol levels that plague so many ex-keto dieters, they will usually be very pleased with their cholesterol levels when they are living the Mediterranean-keto lifestyle. The same applies to their other symptoms.

This isn't a new trend or craze. It's a lifestyle that people in the Mediterranean countries have been living for centuries, and the health benefits are well documented.

If you need to lose weight or are suffering from ailments, an illness, or a disease, then I strongly suggest that you start with the keto diet (part 1 of this book) and then roll that into the Mediterranean-keto lifestyle (part 2). Follow these with recipes and meal planning (part 3), and you are on your way! If you are pleased with your weight and health, feel free to head directly into the Mediterranean-keto lifestyle.

Amazingly the Mediterranean-keto lifestyle is a weight loss plan, a treatment plan, and a prevention plan—it helps prevent almost all the diseases and cancers that plague society—all rolled into one. If you want these health options, there is none better.

This is a disease-stopping, weight-reduction, healthy lifestyle, but don't rush unless you want to or have to. Take it at the pace that suits you and your family the best. The end goal is a healthy lifestyle that you enjoy for years to come.

I'll see you there.

Chapter 1

THE NORM—AND WHY WE ARE HERE

WHEN IT COMES to food, we typically do what we are told, eat what's put in front of us, follow the food recommendations of the US Department of Agriculture (USDA), listen to our doctors, and let society dictate our eating habits. We basically follow along.

Some will argue, "That's not true. I'm not controlled by anyone. I eat whatever I want." That is also true—and also part of the problem!

You see, as a whole, we in the Western world (the United States, in particular) eat whatever we want, then go to doctors and expect them to fix what ails us. But there is no magic pill that makes us lose weight, much less stems the tide of all the sicknesses and diseases that come as a result of what we put in our mouths.

The government is of little to no help either. Take a look at the US dietary guidelines, and you will see it is recommended that carbohydrates make up 45–65 percent of our calories per day.[1] If we eat 2,000 calories a day on average, that means 900–1,300 calories, or 225–325 grams, should be from carbs every day. No wonder we are fat!

We eat on average 133 pounds of flour per person per year,[2] which translates into about 1.3 cups of flour per person per day. That's a lot of carbohydrates, which then turn into sugar when our bodies use it for fuel. The fact is, the sugar and corresponding insulin spikes in the body with processed carbs, and many non-processed ones, are similar to straight sugar.

As for sugar itself, we eat a lot of it! The average American eats and drinks a total of about 130 pounds of sugar each year.[3] There are about thirty-six tablespoons in one pound of sugar, so that breaks down to almost thirteen tablespoons of sugar each day per person! Most of the sugar is hidden in foods and drinks, but still, is it any wonder that prediabetes, type 2 diabetes, obesity, and insulin resistance numbers are off the charts?

And did you know that our sugar addiction is actually a biological disorder, driven by insulin, appetite hormones, and neurotransmitters that fuel our insatiable food cravings and "affect the same brain pleasure centers as heroin or cocaine"?[4] Not only are the sugars (and carbs) we consume addictive, but they play with our minds, our hormones, and our wallets!

Of course, our expanding waistlines are not solely the result of consuming the daily recommended number of carbs along with lots and lots of sugar, but carbs and sugar play a significant part in our overall weight gain. Don't believe me? The United States is the most overweight industrialized nation in the world.[5] More than 70 percent of the US population over age twenty is considered overweight.[6] In 1960 only 13.4 percent of the US population was obese, and now we are up to over 40 percent.[7] And because obesity is a root cause of many diseases, it would then follow that we would have a dramatic increase in these obesity-related diseases over the past fifty to sixty years. That is precisely what is happening. According to the Centers for Disease Control and Prevention (CDC), more than 10 percent of the US population already has full-blown type 2 diabetes and almost 35 percent of those over age eighteen have prediabetes.[8] That means we are almost to 50 percent of the US population being prediabetic or type 2 diabetic! In fact, we may have already crossed that point, as that stat is already being reported.[9]

Those high blood-sugar levels also affect our memory. One ten-year study of over 5,100 people found that those with high blood sugar had faster rates of cognitive decline than those with normal blood-sugar levels.[10] Diabetics have almost twice the risk of developing dementia.[11]

But that is not all. High glucose and high insulin levels are also predictors of cancer and cancer-related death.[12] Over time, obesity leads to insulin resistance, which is usually a root cause of heart disease, obesity, diabetes, cancer, and dementia.[13] A study found that only 12 percent of Americans are metabolically healthy, meaning that 88 percent have either insulin resistance or significant risk factors for it.[14]

These foods we eat of our own free will—all readily available, approved by the US Food and Drug Administration (FDA), and USDA recommended—also cause inflammation, and we now know that inflammation is the source of virtually all chronic diseases. Those nasty chronic diseases include autoimmune diseases, cardiovascular disease, arthritis, cancer, Alzheimer's disease, and Parkinson's disease.

As expected, there has been a steady rise in the frequency of auto-immune diseases in the last several decades.[15] Today around fifty million Americans have an autoimmune condition,[16] millions more are on the autoimmune-inflammation spectrum, there is a heart attack every thirty-four seconds,[17] and 40.14 percent of men and 38.7 percent of women get cancer.[18]

IT'S A FACT

The average American consumes 130 pounds of sugar each year, about 3,550 pounds in a lifetime.[19]

Cardiovascular disease, which kills more people than all forms of cancer combined,[20] happens to be the costliest killer as well. The American Heart Association (AHA) states that heart disease is increasing and predicts that 45 percent of the US population will have at least one issue related to the disease by 2035, with the associated costs expected to double, from $555 billion in 2016 to $1.1 trillion in 2035.[21] The AHA noted that unfortunately other risk factors, such as obesity, poor diet, high blood pressure, and type 2 diabetes, are on the rise.[22] Not only are Americans not getting the message about heart disease, but they are not getting the message about what they should eat and drink.

Combining obesity with inflammation is like tying a brick to a paper airplane in a rainstorm and expecting it to fly. It is doubly impossible.

Doctors do their best to stand in the gap. They usually recommend more exercise, fewer sweets, and more fruits and vegetables. That's good advice. In fact, researchers estimate that if we would just eat ten servings of fruits and vegetables a day (which is about 800 grams, or 28 ounces), then close to 7.8 million deaths worldwide could be prevented.[23]

Do you think this is happening? Of course not. Millions of lives and billions of dollars could be saved by people simply eating more fruits and vegetables. Doing so reduces the risk of virtually everything, from type 2 diabetes and obesity to cardiovascular disease and some types of cancer. Approximately 12 percent of US adults meet the American dietary guidelines for fruit consumption (one and a half to two cups per day) and less than 10 percent do so for vegetable consumption (two to three cups a day).[24]

The top fruits, apples and oranges in the form of juice, are both high in fructose (a natural sugar), which also plays into our runaway insulin levels and obesity rates.[25] But we do eat some vegetables. Yes, we do, but mainly potatoes and tomatoes in the form of french fries and pizza![26] When the primary vegetables we do eat have added inflammatory oils, salt, and sugar, you can bet the nutritional value is reduced to almost nothing.

As you would expect with only 10–12 percent of the US population eating their fruits and vegetables, we are low in vitally important vitamins and minerals.

- Vitamin K_2: 97 percent of Americans may be low in vitamin K_2.[27]

- Fiber: Virtually none of my patients initially consume enough fiber. This is vital for your body's health at many levels, and I will write more about fiber later, but I estimate that 95 percent of all Americans are low in fiber. That estimate holds true, for research shows that only 5 percent of Americans consume enough fiber.[28]

- Omega-3: 90 percent of Americans have insufficient levels of omega-3 fats.[29]

- Potassium: 97 percent of American adults are deficient in potassium.[30] Many fruits and vegetables have abundant potassium.

- Vitamin A: 51 percent of American adults are deficient in vitamin A.[31]

- Vitamin C: 43 percent of American adults are deficient in vitamin C.[32]

- Magnesium: 50 percent of Americans are deficient in magnesium.[33]

- Vitamin D: Approximately 42 percent are deficient in vitamin D, and that increases to over 70 percent in older adults.[34]

- Calcium: One survey found that about 10 percent of girls age fourteen to eighteen, less than 10 percent of women over age fifty, 22 percent of boys age nine to thirteen, and 22 percent of men age fifty-one to seventy took in enough calcium.[35]

The list of deficiencies is daunting, but even more disturbing is that each nutrient is supposed to play a role in the body to protect us from the very things that plague us. We desperately need what we are not getting.

To add insult to injury, while our bodies are deficient in so many vitamins and minerals, we throw a host of other things into our bodies that cause untold damage. From fake sugars to genetically modified organism (GMO) crops to processed meats to growth hormones to herbicides to pesticides to inflammatory oils to high-fructose corn syrup to refined flour to packaged food, we keep making things worse.

One small example is high-fructose corn syrup. This sweetener is used in countless items in our grocery stores, including bread, ketchup, cereal, salad dressing, and cough medicine. High-fructose corn syrup is what is called an obesogen, which is a fancy word for a chemical that makes us fat.[36] This man-made sweetener plays with the hormones in our guts and brains, making us crave more food even when we don't need it.

Interestingly, regular sugar is 50:50 fructose to glucose, but high-fructose corn syrup is 55:45 or even 75:25 fructose to glucose, which means it is sweeter (and more addictive), not to mention cheap (from corn stalks) to make.[37] Yes, we know high-fructose corn syrup is not good for us, yet it's in foods all around us. (Ask yourself, If it's cheap and addictive, why would they stop using it?)

But that is just one example. We could rail against something else, such as fake sugars and how they are bad for your brain, contribute to obesity and belly fat, and are very addictive, but that's just another example of the same.[38]

You can look online at how unhealthy certain chemicals or processes or ingredients are and how research has shown them to be cancer causing or fat inducing or plaque forming or insulin raising or memory impairing, but that doesn't stop them from being in the foods we eat! That's the norm in the United States. That's why we are here. And if you follow the norm and the national averages, then you can expect the nation's health averages as well.

Thankfully food is medicine, and that means by eating the right foods, we can usually reverse or improve virtually everything that ails us. And long term those good foods will also prevent sickness and disease.

That is exciting!

Chapter 2

YOU CAN TAKE CHARGE
OF YOUR HEALTH

DID YOU KNOW that about 75 percent of longevity is the result of your own choices (that includes foods you eat, stress, sleep, exercise, and exposure to toxins) rather than your genes?[1] Odds are it's not in your genes, and that is *great* news!

Combine that reality with the fact that the right foods can reverse, prevent, and cure most of what plagues (or scares) you, and you have a very bright future. So what is your motivation for taking stock of your health?

- Is your goal to lose weight?

- Do you have a family history that concerns you?

- Are you currently suffering from a sickness or disease?

- Are family members dying early of disease?

- Are family members suffering from dementia and ending up in nursing homes?

Unfortunately, if you have a strong family history of Alzheimer's, diabetes, dementia, heart disease, cancer, insulin resistance, or another such disease, you are really signing up for it with the standard American diet. In fact, if you have prediabetes, diabetes, or insulin resistance, you have almost double the risk of developing dementia.[2] And if your parents had it, you need to change your diet right away.

One recent patient suffered from moderate dementia. I told her family, "Dementia can sometimes be reversed through diet, lifestyle, and supplements if we start when the symptoms are mild to moderate. I've done it many times."

The family was encouraged but naturally hesitant to get too hopeful. They were about to take her out of her house and put her in a nursing home for fear that she might forget to turn off the stove or wander away. She had already been forced to quit her part-time job because the details were too much for her.

We started her immediately on a healthy keto diet, which for her meant revising her eating habits entirely. Her family helped, and within a few months she was thinking more clearly, talking more to her adult children, engaging with the grandchildren, and even doing light exercise, such as walking in her neighborhood. Six months later she started working part-time!

Needless to say, her family was both thankful and amazed, but such turnarounds happen all the time. Had her dementia been more advanced, the keto diet would still have helped but it would have probably been too late to reverse all the symptoms.

Also, many patients on a keto diet have high cholesterol levels, and their doctors are prescribing statin medications that may be impairing their memory.

There are over one hundred autoimmune diseases that can often be treated and many times be reversed by changing to a keto diet. The same is true with people losing weight; keeping the weight off; healing a leaky gut; restoring a fatty liver; getting rid of acid reflux; preventing or fighting cancer; lowering high blood-sugar levels; stopping seizures; beating polycystic ovary syndrome (PCOS), small-intestinal bacterial overgrowth (SIBO), and IBS; and so much more.[3] The success stories are endless.

It works because the healthy keto diet usually slows or stops inflammation, heals the gut, feeds the brain, enhances weight loss, lowers insulin levels, reverses insulin resistance, balances sugars, helps prevent plaque buildup, and lowers cholesterol, to name just a few of the benefits to your body. And all of that fuels hope, fresh vision, and new dreams! Life is meant to be lived to the fullest, but it's hard to do so when health problems are staring you right in the face.

If you are looking to lose weight, so is most of the US population! According to the CDC, 73.6 percent of American adults are overweight.[4] That is a great reason to take stock of what you're eating.

INTERNAL MOTIVATION

Four basic things protect us from heart disease, cancer, diabetes, and Alzheimer's. Those are having a healthy diet, not being overweight, exercising about two and a half hours a week, and not smoking. Widespread adoption of these four things would result in a 93 percent decrease in type 2 diabetes cases, an 81 percent decrease in heart attacks, a 50 percent decrease in the number of strokes, and a 36 percent decrease in the incidence of cancer.[5]

One great thing about the keto diet is that it is a weight loss program that increases your metabolism. Instead of starving yourself and slowing down your metabolism, the keto diet actually revs up your engines. And with a higher metabolism, you naturally burn more fat.

Not long ago I had a woman come into my office who was frustrated with her current weight loss efforts. "I've tried all the diets," she exclaimed. "Nothing works. I'm hungrier than ever."

Being hungry usually results in more weight gain, and she admitted that she had actually gained more weight after she enrolled in a local gym! I listened to her situation, discussed her health concerns, and then laid out the science behind the keto diet. She immediately adjusted her diet and kept up her exercise routine, and long story made short, the fat melted off!

She had over one hundred pounds that she wanted to lose, but most people have a spare twenty to fifty pounds they want to lose.

Whatever your motivating reason for pursuing better health, I trust that it is also strong enough to keep you moving forward. As you well know, when it comes to people's health and living a long-term healthy lifestyle, many will start but few will stick with it long enough to really enjoy its benefits.

May the *why* that motivates you be so invigorating that it propels you to achieve your health, longevity, fitness, and weight goals!

You can achieve your healthy lifestyle goals and dreams. Let's do this together.

PART I
THE INS AND OUTS OF KETO

Part 1 explains the ins and outs of the keto diet,
including the many health benefits that come as a
direct result. For most people it will make sense that
they begin right here, but some will want to jump
to part 2. Whatever your motivation is to be healthy
and establish a healthy lifestyle, I commend you.
Stick with it! You are going to love the end result.

Chapter 3

WHAT IS A KETO DIET?

ABOUT ONE HUNDRED years ago doctors at Johns Hopkins University and the Mayo Clinic were given the arduous task of trying to treat patients who suffered from seizures and diabetes. They tested different diets and found that when they reduced carbohydrate intake to almost zero, patients went into ketosis, seizures usually stopped, and blood-sugar levels usually normalized.[1]

Was that the beginning of the keto diet? Not at all. You see, our bodies are used to being in ketosis. As nursing babies, we relied on the fat in our mothers' breast milk for our energy and development. We were in ketosis! And then we slowly transitioned off of it as we began to eat carbs and sugars.[2]

You might be wondering what ketosis is. When you were a baby and your body was burning fat for energy, you were in ketosis. As an adult it's the exact same thing. When you are burning fat for energy, you are in ketosis.

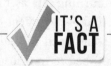

IT'S A FACT

Ketosis is the safe and natural state where your body burns fat for fuel rather than the usual glucose (a sugar in your cells).

Besides being in ketosis for your first year of life, you come pretty close to ketosis whenever you fast or go without food for twelve to fourteen hours between meals (such as eating dinner at 6:00 or 7:00 p.m. and then eating breakfast at 7:00 or 8:00 a.m.).

WHAT EXACTLY IS A KETO DIET?

You know what ketosis is. And you know (from chapter 1) that the normal American diet is a high-carbohydrate diet. After all, that is what the US dietary guidelines recommend, with carbs making up 45–65 percent of our daily intake![3]

These carbs—whether from grains, breads, corn, rice, beans, fruits, potatoes, juices, sugar, pasta, cereals, crackers, sodas, or something else—are turned into glucose in our bodies to be burned as fuel. Extra glucose is stored in your muscles and liver as glycogen and in your liver, belly, hips, and thighs as fat. It's simply what your body does.

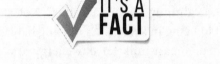

The high amounts of carbs and sugars in the typical American diet usually cause excess fat, less muscle, and insulin resistance. A keto diet will break that, and you usually lose weight, gain muscle, prevent diabetes, and reverse insulin resistance.

So when exactly does this ketosis happen? It can only happen when you lower your carb intake enough for your body to shift from burning sugars as fuel to burning fats as fuel. For most people that number is going to be around 5–15 percent of their daily food intake coming from carbs. Yes, some need to dial that number back even further (less than 5 percent) before they lose weight, and it may take anywhere from two days to eight weeks to enter ketosis.

When carbs are reduced to below whatever your carb threshold is, you naturally start to lose weight. And don't worry, carbs are not required to live. You need proteins and fats to survive, but technically carbs are not required to sustain life.

I have had people tell me there is no way they can survive without their bread or soda or chips or candy or ice cream, but they do. In fact, once they have gone without their must-have carbs and their bodies have adjusted to burning fat rather than glucose, they often tell me, "I don't crave it anymore. In fact, I don't even want it."

The usual goal of most people on a keto diet is to lose weight, and when you reduce your carbohydrate intake to 5–15 percent of your calorie intake, your metabolism will eventually shift from glucose burning to fat burning. Patients who are not insulin resistant, prediabetic, or diabetic can usually shift into ketosis in two to seven days. For those who are insulin resistant, prediabetic, or diabetic, it may take four to eight weeks to enter ketosis, or fat burning.

Reducing your daily carbs is the biggest part of the equation, and that will do wonders to anyone's health. The other half of the equation includes healthy fats and proteins.

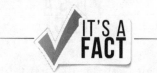

Carbage is a term used to describe highly processed carbohydrates that we consume. Eating these foods is similar to putting garbage into our bodies (hence the name); we are essentially consuming sugar, which invites almost all disease into our bodies.

Not only is the keto diet low-carb; it is also a high-fat, moderate-protein diet. It looks like this:

- Low-carb (5–15 percent), from healthy carbs (e.g., green vegetables, salads, nuts, seeds, non-starchy vegetables, or others)

- High fat (60–75 percent), from healthy fats (e.g., olive oil, avocado oil, omega-3—such as fish oil, nuts, small amounts of cheese, butter, cream, and so on)

- Moderate protein (15–25 percent), from healthy proteins
  (e.g., wild fish, organic pastured eggs, grass-fed meats,
  pastured chicken and turkey, and so on)

Admittedly this is quite a shift for most people. After all, it goes against the US dietary guidelines and our national habits, family culture, restaurant menus, food marketing campaigns, and personal preferences. But when you reduce carbohydrate intake to 5–15 percent, your body is going to go looking for fuel to burn. As a result, it burns fat, and the first fat to burn is usually belly fat. Nobody complains about that!

IT'S A
FACT

When you first get into ketosis, the first fat to burn off is usually belly fat.

Not only do the high-fat and moderate-protein parts of the keto equation help your body burn fat more efficiently, but they also help keep you from being hungry, give you the energy you need, and restore your body.

We will look in greater detail at the many benefits of the keto diet in the next chapter, but here is a quick snapshot that excites most people. A healthy keto diet

- promotes weight loss (an average of one to two pounds
  of fat per week)

- often burns belly fat first

- reduces appetite

- increases energy

- increases metabolism

- promotes greater mental clarity (focus)

- reduces brain fog

- reduces the need for afternoon naps

- virtually eliminates sugar spikes or crashes

- keeps food cravings under control

- reduces inflammation, which usually means less pain.

We are taught that our bodies are mostly water, but let's say you remove all the water. Do you know what remains? Interestingly well over half your solid body matter is fat, a smaller amount is protein, and only about 1 percent is made up of carbs, similar to the keto diet!

Here's another interesting fact: about 60 percent of your brain and nervous system is made of fat.[4] So all those low-fat diets and low-fat recommendations are starving your already-hungry body, especially your brain. And that's one of the reasons the keto diet with 70 percent healthy fat is so incredibly healthy and beneficial in treating brain-related diseases.

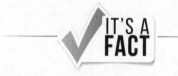

IT'S A
FACT

Your brain is the fattiest organ in your body, and 25 percent of your body's cholesterol is in your brain. Eating cholesterol and fat feeds your brain, which means going low fat and low cholesterol is actually starving your brain.[5]

Yet another keto-related detail is that the glucose your body usually burns has a currency, or value. Energy burned in the cells is measured in adenosine triphosphate (ATP) molecules. One unit of glucose produces thirty-six ATP molecules, while one unit of fat produces over twice that amount. That simply means that burning fat gives you twice as much energy as burning sugar does.[6] All this is further evidence that getting your body into ketosis, where you are using fat rather than glucose for fuel, is a good thing!

STAY FOCUSED ON YOUR GOAL

Your goal as you get on the keto diet is to focus on consuming healthy fats (around 70 percent of your diet) and moderate proteins (15–25 percent) and to keep your carbs low (5–15 percent). How long will it take for your body to shift from burning glucose to burning fat for fuel? It varies per person, depending on age; health; eating habits; if you are insulin resistant, prediabetic, or diabetic; exercise habits; and so on, but I tell patients that it can be as little as a few days to as long as a month or two.

On average, I would say it takes about two to seven days for my healthier patients. But for patients who are insulin resistant, prediabetic, or diabetic, it usually takes four to eight weeks, and that's usually about right for heavier, older patients. Later we'll talk about supplements that help you enter ketosis within one hour. But the point is, keep going, and you will get there. Countless health benefits await!

Chapter 4

THE MANY HEALTH BENEFITS OF A KETO DIET

Y OU WILL LOVE the benefits that come from a keto diet. The great news, which I enjoy telling people, is that these benefits can last a lifetime. With keto as a lifestyle (part 2 of this book), you and your family can enjoy these benefits forever.

Amazingly, and very thankfully, the keto diet addresses many of today's toughest health issues, which means this can be both a treatment plan and a prevention plan. It depends on where you are and what you need, but either way you win!

The following is a highly abbreviated explanation of just sixteen of the many health benefits of a keto diet.

BENEFIT 1: BURNS FAT INSTEAD OF SUGAR

Burning fat is far more efficient than burning sugar for fuel. This is better for your metabolism, helping you lose weight more quickly. It's like converting your metabolism from a gas-burning engine to a hybrid engine, which is far more efficient.[1] (More on this in chapter 7.)

BENEFIT 2: SNUFFS OUT INFLAMMATION AND DECREASES ARTHRITIS PAIN

Inflammation is a root cause of virtually every chronic disease. (That includes most cardiovascular diseases, arthritis, most cancers, autoimmune diseases, IBS, psoriasis, most lung diseases, Alzheimer's disease, Parkinson's disease, gum disease, depression, etc.) A keto diet helps snuff out inflammation.[2] Inflammatory foods include polyunsaturated fats, such as soybean oil and corn oil, especially when used to deep-fry; trans fats, such as margarine; excessive sugars, carbs, and starches, especially when processed; and usually gluten and conventional dairy as well as other foods. It's a vicious cycle. The more sugar, carbs, and starches you consume, the higher your insulin level rises. Excessive insulin causes more fat storage and more inflammation and unleashes a ravenous appetite, and the cycle continues.

For many with arthritis, a healthy keto diet with minimal or no dairy is usually pain relieving. One of my older patients was about eighty years old and suffered severely from arthritis, especially in his knees and hands. He couldn't even clap his hands because of pain and swelling, much less squat down to tie his shoes. He went on a keto diet without dairy and nightshades (tomatoes, potatoes, peppers, eggplant, or paprika) and six months later came in for an appointment. When I saw him, he didn't shake my hand as expected. Instead, he clapped his hands together several times and did ten squats all the way to the ground! He used to wince in pain while he walked, and now he was bouncing around my office like a spry young man. The healthy keto diet removed his inflammation, and he was incredibly thankful to be pain-free and active again.

BENEFIT 3: LOWERS INSULIN LEVELS, HELPS CONTROL BLOOD SUGAR, AND SOMETIMES REVERSES TYPE 2 DIABETES

The normal cycle of a high-carb diet requires the body to pump out insulin to manage and lower the sugar so the body can convert the sugar to energy and fat. Over time, and with so much insulin being pumped out, the cell's insulin receptors become insulin resistant and less efficient, which requires more insulin to do the same task, and the blood sugar begins to rise higher and higher.[3] This ever-increasing inefficiency is called insulin resistance. The number one way to lower blood-sugar levels (and prevent and/or treat type 2 diabetes and pre-diabetes) is to restrict carbs and increase fat intake, which is exactly what a keto diet does.[4] High insulin levels also cause inflammation. A keto diet reduces insulin levels and inflammation and improves insulin receptor sensitivity.[5]

WHAT CAUSES TYPE 2 DIABETES?

Over time our bodies grow tired of the high amount of insulin required to manage a high-carbohydrate diet. In response our cells reduce their number of insulin-sensitive receptors. Think of it like a house with many doors, and insulin is the only substance that opens those doors and lets glucose in. But too much insulin causes many of these doors to be boarded up from the inside. That means insulin and glucose pile up outside, in our blood, and all that sugar in the bloodstream causes inflammation. This wears away at our arteries and organs and causes aging. Our pancreas tries to account for the closed doors by pumping out even more insulin to remove the extra glucose. At that point we have type 2 diabetes! (This same process also causes heart disease.) In one study people with type 2 diabetes went on a keto diet for twenty-four weeks. The results were astounding: 95 percent had better glucose levels and were able to reduce the dosage of diabetes medications or even quit taking them entirely.[6]

BENEFIT 4: CONTROLS APPETITE HORMONES

High insulin levels cause the body to store calories in the form of fat. Leptin, the hormone that controls appetite, is also affected by insulin. When insulin resistant, the body no longer responds to leptin signals, so figuratively speaking, the you-are-full signal is not flashing, and you naturally eat more and gain weight, and diabetes and obesity usually follow.[7] This is also called leptin resistance. Decreasing sugars, carbs, and starches dramatically; increasing exercise; getting adequate sleep; and consuming fish and fish oils regularly can improve leptin sensitivity, which helps control one's appetite. The reduction in the fat-storage hormone (insulin) makes a huge difference in losing weight and keeping weight off. This alone is the reason many people stay on the keto diet, for it controls appetite and prevents the typical weight gain that people experience on other dieting methods. (More on this in chapter 7.)

BENEFIT 5: IMPROVES/CURES ACID REFLUX

Acid reflux, or gastroesophageal reflux disease (GERD), usually experienced as heartburn, is most often caused by pressure on the diaphragm from belly fat or pregnancy. Medications (sometimes with adverse side effects) can treat acid reflux symptoms but not cure it. I have found the most common cure of acid reflux is simply losing weight in the abdomen, and the keto diet usually burns belly fat. It is estimated that the health care cost of treating GERD is around ten billion dollars a year.[8] The condition is mostly the result of eating the typical American diet of whole grains and sugars, but on a keto diet, without all the carbohydrates, GERD usually improves or goes away completely.

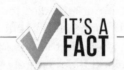

Foods that often make acid reflux (GERD) worse include alcohol, chocolate, peppermint, spearmint, and caffeine.

BENEFIT 6: REDUCES PLAQUE IN ARTERIES

Nearly 80 percent of heart attacks, strokes, or sudden cardiac deaths are from small areas of unstable plaque on the blood vessel lining (that are 20–40 percent blocked with plaque) that burst like a pimple. Inflammation is the primary reason for these plaque-rupturing lesions on the artery lining. A sudden rupture of plaque releases chemicals into the bloodstream, which causes blood to clot, and you've got blocked blood flow! In an artery to your heart, that's a heart attack; in your brain, that's a stroke. Lowering blood-sugar levels, blood pressure, inflammation, and cholesterol levels usually prevents plaque growth and helps stabilize plaque, making it less likely to rupture.[9] And this is exactly what this healthy keto diet does.

BENEFIT 7: DECREASES ALZHEIMER'S RISK

Our bodies have an insulin-degrading enzyme that regulates the level of insulin by degrading it, or breaking it down. This same enzyme also breaks down an inflammatory protein (beta-amyloid) and an amyloid precursor protein (APP), which are directly associated with Alzheimer's disease. When there is excess insulin in our bodies, this enzyme breaks down insulin first, which eventually leads to a buildup of beta-amyloid and APP. This is just another reason prediabetics and diabetics are programming themselves for Alzheimer's disease.[10]

BENEFIT 8: USUALLY LOWERS CHOLESTEROL AND TRIGLYCERIDE LEVELS AND HELPS PREVENT HEART DISEASE

Because a keto diet lowers insulin levels, that means your body stores less fat. Triglyceride levels usually fall dramatically, and bad, low-density lipoprotein (LDL) cholesterol usually falls—unless you are consuming excessive amounts of saturated fats, including butter, cream, cheese, coconut oil, medium-chain triglyceride (MCT) oil, ghee, fried foods, and fatty meats, which can raise cholesterol levels—while good, high-density lipoprotein (HDL) cholesterol usually rises.[11] This in turn usually reduces the risk of heart attack and stroke.

Most heart disease (the biggest killer in the world) is caused by inflammation and insulin resistance, prediabetes, or type 2 diabetes, all of which are addressed on a keto diet. When there is inflammation in the body (which occurs on the typical American diet), the arteries and arterioles eventually form plaque, which accumulates, setting the stage for heart disease.

BENEFIT 9: FIGHTS CANCER

Cancer cells usually depend on sugar to survive, but a keto diet usually helps starve the cancer cells. Without sugar those cancer cells usually cannot live, much less spread or multiply. A keto diet is the absolute best diet for cancer. Neurologist Thomas Seyfried calls the keto diet and other metabolic strategies "the most cost-effective, nontoxic approach to cancer prevention and management."[12] It was discovered back in the 1920s by Dr. Otto Warburg that cancer cells consume more glucose than normal cells. If you remove sugar, or carbs that turn to sugar in the body, cancer cells may die.[13]

BENEFIT 10: FUELS THE BRAIN

The brain relies on sufficient amounts of the right types of fat for fuel and energy. Neurological disorders can occur when the brain is starved of certain fats. The ketones generated while in ketosis give the brain even more energy than a typical glucose-derived diet can, and this has been found to improve cognitive function in Alzheimer's patients,[14] decrease symptoms by 43 percent in Parkinson's patients after just a month,[15] and improve learning abilities and social skills in autistic children.[16] A keto diet may even protect you from Alzheimer's, Parkinson's, epilepsy, headaches, brain injuries, sleep disorders, and more.[17]

Foods that your brain and liver really enjoy include coffee (without cream and sugar), fish oil (omega-3), walnuts, avocado, and high-phenolic olive oil.

BENEFIT 11: LOWERS BLOOD PRESSURE

One very natural benefit of the keto diet is weight loss, which usually helps lower blood pressure immediately by promoting the loss of sodium. High insulin levels promote sodium retention, and when patients start a keto diet, their insulin levels often drop drastically, they lose sodium, and usually their blood pressure lowers as well. With the keto diet, lowering blood pressure is relatively easy; no medications are required, and generally the more weight someone loses, the lower the blood pressure drops. Blood pressure usually decreases as belly fat decreases. Belly fat produces a lot of C-reactive protein, which is an inflammatory marker and constricts the arteries.

BENEFIT 12: HELPS A FATTY LIVER

Fatty liver disease, which affects about a third (one hundred million!) of Americans, may eventually lead to liver failure. It is not alcohol related, and those who are obese, are sedentary, or consume a highly processed diet are most likely to have a fatty liver.[18] There is no medical treatment for it yet, but a healthy keto diet with more olive oil and avocado oil, fewer saturated fats, and regular exercise is the best way to prevent or reverse liver disease.[19] Excessive sugar, high-fructose corn syrup, sodas, juices (full of fructose), honey, syrup, agave nectar, and excessive sweet fruits are fuel in this fatty liver epidemic.

BENEFIT 13: IMPROVES/CURES PCOS

For the women who suffer from polycystic ovary syndrome (PCOS), there is hope! The cause of PCOS is an imbalance of hormones, with too much luteinizing hormone (LH) and too little follicle-stimulating hormone (FSH), which prevents ovulation. (The eggs remain in the ovaries and form small cysts.) Women with PCOS usually have excessive androgens, resulting in masculinizing effects and insulin resistance. The condition usually only worsens over time, with weight gain, male-pattern hair growth, belly fat, fatty liver, and hormone imbalance. The keto diet breaks this cycle, burns fat, alleviates insulin resistance, and helps balance the sex hormones.

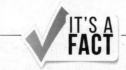
IT'S A FACT

If you have type 1 diabetes, a healthy keto diet can help you lose weight and control blood-sugar levels, but you will need to eat more than 50 grams of carbs per day to prevent ketoacidosis, and you need to continue your insulin, but your doctor will usually need to adjust your insulin dosage to a lower dose. I suggest that you go directly to the Mediterranean-keto lifestyle (part 2). You get the same health benefits, and the carb intake is higher, which is important for anyone with type 1 diabetes. Many of my type 1 diabetics consume 75–100 grams of carbs per day.

BENEFIT 14: SLOWS DOWN THE AGING PROCESS

Advanced glycation end products (AGEs) occur when proteins or fats become glycated from exposure to sugar. They are also found in some of the foods. These AGEs actually age you when proteins and fats combine with the sugar in your bloodstream. AGEs accumulate and cause even more inflammation and accelerate aging. They are linked to diabetes, heart disease, and Alzheimer's disease.[20] By lowering one's sugar, the keto diet also lowers AGEs. A keto diet drastically reduces or removes inflammation from the body, which is known to cause plaque in the arteries, damage organs, and bring about age-related sicknesses and disease. It also drastically lowers blood-sugar levels, which is also an aging accelerator. Slowing down the aging of your body is possible with a keto diet because it addresses the root causes of aging.[21]

There are countless more benefits to a keto diet than those listed here. If you are fighting a sickness or disease, the odds are very high that a keto diet will help relieve the symptoms and in many cases restore your body to good health.

Over the years, I have seen every single one of these benefits in my patients. For many, it was the difference between life and death, between a downward slide to poor health and an upward surge to freedom, or between sadness and happiness.

You get to choose. With these benefits and the keto diet as the foundation, your health is on the right track. For more information on the benefits of the keto diet, refer to my book *Dr. Colbert's Keto Zone Diet*.

Chapter 5

THREE ADDITIONS TO MAKE A KETO DIET EVEN HEALTHIER

A KETO DIET HAS so many great health benefits, as the previous chapter outlined, that it's attractive and beneficial to everyone. Who doesn't want to slow down the aging process, lose weight, get healthy, and avoid diseases?

As a doctor, I recommend a healthy keto diet to my patients. As someone who wants to stay healthy, control my weight, and prevent the sicknesses and diseases that plague most Americans, I do what I recommend.

I started on the keto diet, and when my weight was where I wanted it to be, I shifted over to a Mediterranean-keto lifestyle. We will discuss all of this—the keto-diet-to-Mediterranean-keto-lifestyle shift—in the coming chapters and show you how to do the same. One feeds right into the other. The Mediterranean-keto lifestyle is a natural next step after the keto diet, and it is one that you will enjoy.

As you begin the keto diet journey, it is vitally important that you avoid the pitfalls that others on a keto diet have encountered. If we can learn from someone else's mistakes, we certainly should.

After using and researching a keto diet and recommending it to my patients for many years, I began to see certain gaps within the keto diet that need to be filled. These gaps are divided into separate categories: what we need *more* of and what we need *less* of. (This chapter breaks down what you need more of. The next chapter breaks down what you should avoid.)

The top three vitally important additions to any keto diet are

1. more vegetables

2. more fiber

3. more omega-3.

Even with the countless benefits and amazing success stories from a keto diet, these big issues must be addressed by each of us if we want to safely maximize a keto diet and move confidently and knowledgeably into a Mediterranean-keto lifestyle.

1. VEGETABLES—YOU NEED TO EAT MORE!

Believe it or not, people on a standard keto diet do not eat enough veggies.[1] You would think that they, of all people, would be aware of the need for vegetables, but on average most keto dieters are woefully short on their vegetable intake.

We all need 4–9 cups per day of low-sugar, non-starchy vegetables. (For example, a potato is very starchy, as is a sweet potato, corn, or peas.) I always recommend these low-starch, low-sugar veggies (and yes, a few are technically fruits):

- avocados
- cabbage
- broccoli
- celery
- lettuce
- spinach
- artichokes
- bean sprouts
- brussels sprouts
- radishes
- cauliflower
- greens (kale, collard, mustard)

- asparagus

- garlic

- mushrooms

- onions (of all sorts)

- spaghetti squash and summer squashes such as yellow squash and zucchini (not winter squashes such as acorn, butternut, buttercup, or pumpkin, which are high in starch)

- peppers (known to cause gut issues, so use sparingly or not at all if your body doesn't like them)

- tomatoes (known to cause gut issues, so use sparingly or not at all if your body doesn't like them)

And with the vegetables, you can eat all you want!

Some vegetables, such as carrots, are higher in sugar than other vegetables. Carrots are fine to eat, but I recommend them in small amounts (a quarter cup or less). On a keto diet you always have to keep in mind the number of daily carbs. If you eat too many carrots, your body will slip right out of ketosis for the day.

Another important factor with vegetables (and fruit) is whether they are toxin-free (organic, natural, and not sprayed with pesticides, insecticides, herbicides, etc.). You may have heard the terms Dirty Dozen and Clean Fifteen. They are two different lists, one with fruits and vegetables that are best to eat organic (to be sure they have no toxins) and the other with nonorganic fruits and vegetables that are fine to eat.

Here is the latest list of Clean Fifteen fruits and vegetables, which you don't need to buy organic:

1. avocados

2. sweet corn (avoid on a keto diet)

3. pineapple (avoid or limit on a keto diet)

4. onions

5. papaya (avoid or limit on a keto diet)

6. frozen sweet peas (avoid on a keto diet)

7. eggplant

8. asparagus

9. broccoli

10. cabbage

11. kiwi (limit on a keto diet)

12. cauliflower

13. mushrooms

14. honeydew melon (avoid or limit on a keto diet)

15. cantaloupe (avoid or limit on a keto diet)[2]

And here is the latest Dirty Dozen list, items that are best to buy organic:

1. strawberries

2. spinach

3. kale, collard, and mustard greens

4. nectarines (avoid or limit on a keto diet)

5. apples (avoid or limit on a keto diet)

6. grapes (avoid or limit on a keto diet)

7. cherries (avoid or limit on a keto diet)

8. peaches (avoid or limit on a keto diet)

9. pears (avoid or limit on a keto diet)

10. bell and hot peppers

11. celery

12. tomatoes[3]

If the sugar content is too high to stay in ketosis, especially with the fruits, you will simply need to consume smaller amounts or wait until you are ready to shift from a strictly keto diet to the Mediterranean-keto lifestyle, where you can eat more healthy fruits that are lower in sugar.

The bottom line is that you need to eat sufficient amounts—4–9 cups per day—of low-sugar, non-starchy vegetables. Trust me, it's easier and more enjoyable than it may sound. The recipes and food plans in the coming pages will help.

2. FIBER—YOU ABSOLUTELY MUST HAVE MORE!

Just as with vegetables, people on a typical keto diet are not getting enough fiber—far from it! And I can't stress it enough: you need more fiber!

As I have already mentioned, very seldom is one of my patients consuming enough fiber. Fiber is vital for our health, yet only 5 percent of Americans consume enough fiber.[4]

Normally when people say they need more fiber in their diets, most people think it's code for being constipated, but fiber is far more than a laxative. Yet constipation is a very serious matter. A lot of my patients (especially those over age seventy) talk a lot about their bowel movements. Strange? Not at all. Constipation usually worsens with age. It's a combination of aging muscles, a lack of water and magnesium, medications (such as antacids), and a low-fiber diet that does it.

In fact, more than forty million adults in the United States (about 16 percent of the population) suffer from chronic constipation (meaning that the constipation lasts for thirty days or more!), which results in almost seven thousand doctor visits and nearly two thousand emergency room visits per day![5]

Interestingly the disease that generates the most gut-related doctor visits is acid reflux. More than sixty million people in the United

States have acid reflux at least once per month, and the usual prescription is an antacid, which contributes directly to constipation.[6]

In case you are wondering just how important it is to get enough fiber in your diet, consider this list, a mere sampling of what fiber can do for you:

- helps you lose weight

- normalizes bowel movements

- decreases inflammation

- makes you feel full longer, thus controlling appetite

- increases insulin sensitivity

- slows digestion

- gives you energy

- lowers bad cholesterol levels (I've seen a 10–20 percent decrease in some of my patients.)

- lowers blood pressure

- improves your metabolism

- lowers blood-sugar levels

- makes your gut happy

- lowers your risk of heart disease, stroke, and obesity

- prevents diverticular disease

- helps lower hemoglobin A1C numbers for diabetics

- eases IBS symptoms

- minimizes hemorrhoids and anal fissures

Are you enjoying these health benefits from fiber? With only 5 percent of Americans getting enough fiber, odds are that you are not! Statistically speaking, the average adult in America is only getting

15 grams of fiber per day. According to the Institute of Medicine, women need 25 grams of fiber per day and men need 38 grams of fiber per day.[7] The USDA recommends less fiber for both men and women over age fifty, but I disagree.[8] We all need fiber, especially as we age. I recommend 30–35 grams of fiber per day, but start low and go slow to avoid bloating and gas.

Where does fiber come from? How much do you need to eat per day to no longer be deficient in fiber? This short list (from the Mayo Clinic) contains several common foods and their fiber content:[9]

Fruits	Serving Size	Total Fiber (grams)*
Raspberries	1 cup	8.0
Pear	1 medium	5.5
Apple, with skin	1 medium	4.5
Banana	1 medium	3.0
Orange	1 medium	3.0
Strawberries	1 cup	3.0

Vegetables	Serving size	Total Fiber (grams)*
Green peas, boiled	1 cup	9.0
Broccoli, boiled	1 cup chopped	5.0
Turnip greens, boiled	1 cup	5.0
Brussels sprouts, boiled	1 cup	4.0
Potato, with skin, baked	1 medium	4.0
Sweet corn, boiled	1 cup	3.5
Cauliflower, raw	1 cup chopped	2.0
Carrot, raw	1 medium	1.5

Legumes, Nuts, and Seeds	Serving Size	Total Fiber (grams)*
Split peas, boiled	1 cup	16.0
Lentils, boiled	1 cup	15.5
Black beans, boiled	1 cup	15.0
Baked beans, canned	1 cup	10.0
Chia seeds	1 ounce	10.0
Almonds	1 ounce (23 nuts)	3.5
Pistachios	1 ounce (49 nuts)	3.0
Sunflower kernels	1 ounce	3.0

*Rounded to the nearest 0.5 gram

Many of these high-fiber foods will not be part of your initial keto diet but will be added later on to the Mediterranean-keto lifestyle, especially the beans, peas, and lentils.

As usual on a keto diet, you have to watch the carbs from these, especially the fruits and beans. But regardless of how much fiber you may plan to eat, I still always recommend that you take plant fiber in the form of psyllium husk powder. It comes from the husks of the seeds from the *Plantago ovata* plant. This source of fiber has zero net carbs, and equally important, it's inexpensive and easy to add to your daily routine. (Refer to appendix A for recommended supplements.)

Psyllium husk powder is a perfect blend of soluble fiber (70 percent) and insoluble fiber (30 percent). The soluble part helps you feel full, aids digestion, benefits your gut, and more, while the insoluble part is what helps keep your bowels happy and regular.

I recommend 2 tablespoons of psyllium husk powder a day, 1 in the morning after breakfast and 1 after dinner or before bed. That will give you, at 5 grams of fiber per tablespoon, 10 grams of fiber each day. You can easily build on that each day to get the necessary fiber into your system. Your body will thank you.

3. OMEGA-3 (FISH OIL)—BOOST YOUR INTAKE!

Things are almost as bad with omega-3 levels as they are with fiber when you look at the normal American adult. I believe the number is even higher, but it is reported that 90 percent of Americans have insufficient levels of omega-3 fats.[10]

Here is a list (in descending order, from most to least) of eleven foods that contain omega-3:

1. chia seeds

2. salmon

3. mackerel

4. cod liver oil

5. walnuts

6. flaxseeds

7. sardines

8. caviar

9. anchovies

10. herring

11. oysters[11]

Unfortunately our typical American diet does not contain enough omega-3 fats in it. I mean, how often do you eat these foods? Salmon and walnuts are common, maybe oysters and flaxseeds, but the typical American is simply not eating these omega-3-rich foods. And since it's not in our usual diet, we are not likely to add it, and we lose.

Here are just a few benefits from omega-3 fats:

- prevent oxidized cholesterol, which forms plaque

- reduce the risk of heart attack and stroke

- decrease inflammation

- boost leptin and reverse leptin resistance
- decreases hunger
- prevent dangerous heart arrhythmias
- lower abnormal triglyceride levels
- prevent blood clots
- improve cognitive function
- reduce joint pain[12]

But there is one newly discovered benefit of omega-3 that changes the game for keto dieters. As you know, keto diets are typically high in saturated fats. I've seen people eat three to six times the daily recommended amount of saturated fats and watch inflammation soar as a result. New research finds that saturated fats also increase inflammation by raising lipopolysaccharides (LPS). (See chapter 6.)

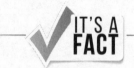

IT'S A
FACT

Saturated fats cause inflammation, especially when eaten with refined carbs or sugar, but we do it all the time:

- bread and butter
- cheese sandwich
- mac and cheese
- hamburger
- ice cream
- hot dog
- BLT

Saturated fats cause inflammation when eaten with refined carbo-hydrates or sugar (e.g., bread and butter) or when you don't get enough omega-3 fats.[13]

Did you catch that? When your body is low in omega-3, the saturated fats that you do eat cause inflammation! Now, I'm not saying to boost your levels of omega-3 so that you can maintain an excessive saturated fat intake. Not at all. The fact is, almost everyone on a keto diet consumes some saturated fat, and if they are not also getting enough omega-3 in their diet, they are letting inflammation in.

KETO BACKWARD

The absolute worst health move is keto dieters returning to the normal high-carb, high-sugar American diet while continuing to eat an excessive amount of saturated fats (e.g., butter, cheese, processed meats).

But there is even more! The omega-3–saturated fat combination is fascinating. When (and only when) your body has sufficient omega-3, the saturated fats that you do eat will actually reduce inflammation by inhibiting genes that produce inflammation, promote the production of other anti-inflammatory agents, lower triglycerides, increase HDL (the good cholesterol), and promote the formation of large, light, fluffy, neutral LDL particles.[14] In short, saturated fats work *for* you rather than *against* you *only* when you have enough omega-3 in your system.

How much omega-3 should you consume per day? Most recommendations are for at least 500 milligrams a day, but your body needs omega-3 desperately, so I suggest doubling that to at least 1,000 milligrams per day. (Personally, I take 2,000 milligrams twice a day.)

For most of us, the only way to get that much omega-3 fat is through a supplement. Virtually all health food and grocery stores have ample omega-3 fish oil options. You want omega-3 that is more eicosapentaenoic acid (EPA) than docosahexaenoic acid (DHA), such as 700 milligrams of EPA and 300 milligrams of DHA or as close to a 2:1 ratio as you can get since a 2:1 EPA-to-DHA ratio seems to address inflammatory risk factors more effectively.[15] If you want to improve brain function, I recommend a fish oil with a higher concentration of DHA and less EPA, or around a 1:1 ratio of EPA to DHA.

The American Heart Association recommends that people with coronary heart disease consume 1,000 milligrams of a combination of EPA and DHA each day.[16] The European Food Safety Authority states that omega-3 supplements can be safely consumed by adults at doses up to 5,000 milligrams per day.[17] From now on, don't let your body run short of omega-3.

There you have it, three of the biggest gaps in a typical keto diet, and I would guess that only a few keto dieters are getting enough of these vital additions.

I cannot emphasize enough just how important these additions are. Add them to your daily routine, for now and for the future. You will be glad you did!

Chapter 6

THREE SUBTRACTIONS TO MAKE A KETO DIET EVEN HEALTHIER

AVOIDING PITFALLS IN a keto diet always means making changes. Sometimes it's addition, as the previous chapter showed, and sometimes it's subtraction, as this chapter will explain.

These subtractions have come after much researching, recommending, and using the keto diet for many years. To make your keto diet even healthier, these three items need to be understood so you'll know which foods to avoid to enjoy good health and longevity:

1. inflammation

2. toxins

3. the APOE4 gene

As with the additions to make to your keto diet, this is all about maximizing your current keto diet as well as preparing for a gradual and successful shift into a Mediterranean-keto lifestyle.

Here is what you need less of in your keto diet:

1. INFLAMMATION—YOU MUST DECREASE IT!

You know by now that a root cause of most chronic diseases is inflammation. You also know that a healthy keto diet is the absolute best way to minimize, even eradicate, inflammation in the body. What I didn't realize was that a regular keto diet can still cause inflammation—usually not near the degree of inflammation that comes with the standard American diet but still enough inflammation to do damage to the body.

How is that possible? The answer is in the food. Typically, people on a keto diet eat too much dairy, meat, and artificial sweeteners. But dairy (like gluten) happens to be one of the most inflammatory foods people can eat, and the high amount of dairy that people eat on a keto diet is what causes inflammation.[1]

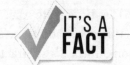

IT'S A
FACT

Ghee (clarified butter) is not as inflammatory because the casein protein has been removed.[2]

Plain and simple, one of the biggest sources of inflammation on a keto diet comes from eating too much dairy. This must be brought under control in order for the keto diet to be as effective and healthy as it's supposed to be.

The most obvious answer is to eat less dairy, and that is exactly what I tell my patients. For example, they can use cheese as a garnish rather than a main part of a meal. Another recommendation is to choose less inflammatory dairy, such as feta cheese (from goat and sheep milk) or ghee (clarified butter). Both do not have the inflammatory proteins that regular cheese and butter have.

Dairy also has saturated fats, but dairy is not the only source of saturated fat. Other foods high in saturated fat include

- beef, pork, lamb, veal, and the skin of poultry

- hot dogs, bologna, salami, sausage, bacon, and pepperoni

- lard, bacon fat, and beef fat

- tropical oils, such as palm, palm kernel, coconut oil, and MCT oil.[3]

Though your body needs some saturated fat, you don't need it in excess. I recommend limiting saturated fats to 7–10 grams per day. The average person on the usual American diet gets 26 grams of saturated fat per day, but the average person on a regular keto diet eating a lot of butter, cheese, cream, coconut oil, bacon, steak, and processed meats might get two or three times that amount, or even ten times that amount!

I have seen many people on a keto diet go hog wild and eat excessive amounts of these foods, putting whole sticks of butter on their food or 5–10 tablespoons or more of cream or butter in their coffee or eating slabs of cheese. That often happens when people are incorrectly told, "Hey, this is keto, so eat as much as you want."

"Everything in moderation" would have been a good warning.

You may be wondering just what it is about saturated fats that causes inflammation. In my *Healthy Gut Zone* book, I explain it in greater detail, but I will summarize here.

You see, your GI tract contains gram-negative bacteria such as E. coli that colonize your colon. When these gram-negative bacteria die, part of the fat component of the cell membrane (lipopolysaccharides, or LPS) causes the inflammatory properties of LPS. LPS is a powerful stimulator of the immune system and promotes inflammation. LPS rides and hides on saturated fats, including butter, cheese, cream, and all the saturated fats listed previously.

Lipopolysaccharides are bad for your gut and gut wall. Other ways to get this LPS into your body include an already leaking gut, infections, overeating, drinking too much alcohol, dysbiosis (excessive amounts of bad bacteria), and smoking.[4] Now, LPS is naturally present in your body and actually helps protect good bacteria in your stomach from being digested by bile, and the LPS is usually cleaned up and excreted by the liver.[5] All this is normal and it happens smoothly.

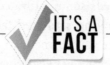

IT'S A FACT

What to remember about LPS:

- The human gut is the biggest source of LPS.
- LPS rides and hides on saturated fats.
- The healthier you are and the healthier your gut is, the lower your LPS levels.
- LPS is the root cause of much inflammation in your body and brain.

However, if your gut is not healthy, these LPS pieces end up passing between the cells of the damaged gut wall and directly into your bloodstream. How do they do it? They "travel through your gut wall and out into the body by riding on and hiding in saturated fats."[6] And that is how saturated fats fuel inflammation while you are busy trying to get healthy on a keto diet. Quite simply, the more saturated fats you have in your body, generally speaking, the more LPS and the more inflammation you will have.

When the LPS pieces get past your gut wall and into your bloodstream, inflammation escalates. A few LPS-related symptoms include

- "fever
- leukocytosis (high [white] blood cell count)
- low iron levels
- blood clotting disorders
- thrombocytopenia (low platelets)
- platelet aggregation."[7]

Studies have found that LPS in your bloodstream can lead to obesity and type 2 diabetes.[8]

LPS levels can be tested, but I don't recommend it for everyone. I usually only test patients who are really sick, and with everyone else I simply suggest that they reduce their saturated fat intake, usually to 10 grams or less per day. If you do want to be tested, ask your doctor to run an LPS blood test for you. It's called Cyrex Laboratories' Array 2—Intestinal Antigenic Permeability Screen. (The test looks for specific antibodies that are signs of LPS in the body, especially the LPS IgA and the LPS IgM antibody tests.)

Here are five easy and practical steps to help lower your LPS levels:

1. Decrease your saturated fats (to less than 10 grams a day for some, less than 7 grams a day for others).

2. Increase your fish oil (omega-3).

3. Increase your fiber intake.

4. Increase your olive oil.

5. Increase your probiotics.

You do not want excess LPS at all in your body since it affects your gut, inflames your body, and will eventually trigger inflammation in your brain. LPS can even increase beta-amyloid in your brain, which is a protein commonly found in the brains of Alzheimer's patients. One of the benefits of a keto diet is that it directly helps lower blood-sugar levels, reduces insulin resistance, and helps clear out beta-amyloid.

Consuming excessive amounts of foods with saturated fats can keep you from getting some of the benefits of a keto diet that you may really want and need. In sum, you can decrease inflammation (and help your gut, brain, and overall health) by decreasing your saturated fat intake.

2. TOXINS—AVOID THEM!

Toxins are in many of the foods we eat. Now, I fully understand that when someone says "toxins," a lot of people will hear "conspiracy theorist." But this is your body and your health we are talking about, so you get to decide what you will eat.

Here are some very abbreviated factors to consider:

Toxin: GMO foods

As I explain in my *Healthy Gut Zone* book, genetically modified organism (GMO) foods were FDA approved and introduced in the 1990s to the US food supply (though GMOs are banned in many countries). GMO foods have pesticides, insecticides, and herbicides added to the seeds to harm insects and diseases that eat or attack them while theoretically not hurting the humans who eat the same foods.

Unfortunately we aren't so lucky:

- GMO foods may lower serotonin levels and interfere with thyroid hormone production.[9]

- GMO foods and other plants treated with glyphosate play a big part in the gut issues we face today.[10]

- GMO foods, because of the pesticides, disrupt the balance of good and bad bacteria in the gut, promoting the growth of harmful bacteria rather than the good.[11]

- GMO foods interfere with your immune system and increase infection rates.[12]

And as you well know, GMOs are everywhere. Some 75 to 80 percent of processed foods contain GMOs, 94 percent of soy is GMOs, over 90 percent of corn is GMOs, and over 90 percent of sugar from sugar beets is GMOs.[13] Most of the canola oil is also genetically modified.

To avoid GMOs, look for organic or non-GMO-marked foods, but that's not the end of it. You see, GMO foods (usually corn, soy, and canola) are used in the beef, poultry, and fish industries and come right back to you in the form of meat, cheese, eggs, and farm-raised fish.

Eating nonorganic, grain-fed conventional meats is a source of inflammation, and it's widely linked to cancer and other health problems.[14]

Toxin: antibiotics

Antibiotics are known to interfere with our guts to kill beneficial bacteria, and they trigger inflammation. Many people take antibiotics a few times each year. But most of the antibiotics used each year in the United States are actually fed to the animals we eat. In fact, 80 percent of antibiotics in the United States are sold to the livestock and poultry industries.[15] As with GMOs, it comes right back to us in the foods we eat, especially beef, pork, chicken, and dairy.

Toxins: HCA and PAH

HCAs (heterocyclic amines) and PAHs (polycyclic aromatic hydrocarbons) are chemicals formed when meat is cooked at high temperatures, such as pan frying or grilling.[16] HCAs and PAHs have been found to cause changes in DNA that may increase the risk of cancer.[17] The primary ways to reduce exposure to HCAs and PAHs are by not overcooking meat and by not eating charred portions. Several studies have also found that marinating meats in wine, vinegar, or herb sauces for several hours (or overnight) before grilling significantly reduces these toxins.[18]

Toxin: obesogens

As their name implies, obesogens are chemicals that make us fat. Some obesogens are endocrine disruptors, meaning they interfere with our hormones.[19] Some obesogens have been linked not only to obesity but also to birth defects, premature puberty in girls, demasculinization in men, breast cancer, and other disorders.[20]

Here are a few common obesogens:

- Bisphenol A (BPA): This synthetic compound is found mostly in plastic food containers, most canned food, and aluminum beverage cans. This is why I do not eat foods out of cans. I choose fresh or frozen veggies and soups in glass jars. Even though there are only small amounts of BPA in these containers, BPA has been found to cause weight gain and obesity. It has even been linked to insulin resistance, diabetes, heart disease, neurological issues, thyroid problems, and cancer.[21]

- Phthalates: These chemicals, which make plastic pliable, are found in plastic water bottles, toys, food containers, cosmetics, shampoos, pharmaceuticals, shower curtains, and paint and affect the hormones in your body.[22] They may cause you to gain weight by interfering with your metabolism.[23] Men are at particular risk of being affected. Studies have found that phthalate exposure in the womb leads to low testosterone levels, undescended testicles, and even genital malformations.[24]

- Artificial sweeteners (aspartame, sucralose, and saccharine): Recommended by many to help with weight loss, artificial sweeteners actually do the opposite. Researchers have discovered that artificial sweeteners can actually increase food consumption by as much as 30 percent.[25] What happens is that the artificial sweeteners, with their much-touted zero carbs, do not raise blood-sugar levels (as normal sugar does), so the brain thinks nothing is there, and the hunger signal is never satisfied.

- MSG: Used to make food taste better, monosodium glutamate (MSG) blocks the "I am full" messages to your brain, increases insulin levels, and causes your blood-sugar levels to drop, making you hungry.[26] MSG has been found to increase the appetite of rats by an incredible 40 percent.[27]

- High-fructose corn syrup: This is another man-made sweetener that plays with the hormones in our guts and brains to make us keep on eating even when we are full.[28] Because high-fructose corn syrup has a 55/45 or even 75/25 fructose/glucose ratio (regular sugar is 50/50 fructose/glucose), it is sweeter and more addictive. Sadly, this sweetener is virtually everywhere: sodas, syrups, canned fruits and veggies, honey, yogurts, agave nectar, peanut butter, condiments, frozen pizza, baked goods, dry pasta, cookies, candy, and much more. Unfortunately this high-fructose corn syrup is converted in the liver directly into fat.[29]

The best way to minimize your contact with most of these obesogens is to try to avoid them. You can't avoid them completely, but you can miss most of them by avoiding foods and beverages stored in plastic containers, avoiding most canned foods and aluminum beverage cans, using stainless steel or quality aluminum water bottles that are not lined with BPA, feeding babies from glass rather than plastic bottles, cooking with cast iron or stainless steel, and using cosmetics and shampoos that are organic and natural.[30]

Toxin: many farm-raised fish

Salmon is one of the most popular fish in the United States, with at least two-thirds of the fresh salmon being farm raised.[31] The salmon raised on these large-scale fish farms are treated with and fed things that will make you second-guess your last fish purchase. You see, these salmon are usually fed food containing a pesticide to kill sea lice (a marine insect that damages the salmon), antibiotics, ground-up chicken bits (feathers, fat, and poop), GMO yeast, soybeans, and a dye to turn the meat pink.[32]

As you can well imagine, in addition to the toxins from the food they eat, some studies have shown these farm-raised salmon have less omega-3 than wild salmon does.[33] For your next salmon purchase, look for wild caught or sustainably harvested farm raised. These will give you a salmon with high omega-3 levels, as it should be.

Toxin: dioxin-like compound—PCB

Fatty meats, farm-raised fish, and most dairy often contain man-made dioxin-like compounds such as PCBs, which are polychlorinated biphenyls and are toxins (banned since 1979 in the United States) that biodegrade by sunlight or microorganisms but collect in the soil and water.[34] Because these PCBs are in the ground and water, they end up in our foods. PCBs are associated with adverse reproductive and developmental effects, increased cancer risk, obesity, type 2 diabetes, and adverse cardiovascular and even neurological effects.[35] The best way to avoid PCBs is to eat more grass-fed, low-fat meats and low-fat wild fish, and less dairy (choose grass-fed, etc.). Fatty meats such as burgers, bacon, and sausage; butter; cheese; cream; and farm-raised fish contain PCBs, toxins that are stored in fatty tissue and accumulate in the body. That is why it is so important to minimize saturated fats to reduce our exposure to PCBs.

3. APOE4 GENE—BE SAFE!

As I mentioned earlier, 75 percent of our longevity is the result of our own choices (that includes foods we eat, stress, sleep, exercise, and exposure to toxins) rather than our genes.[36] That is great news and should be something we are thankful for on a daily basis.

One gene that plays a part in everyone's health puzzle is the APOE gene. It's relevant when we discuss a keto diet, saturated fats, Alzheimer's disease, and alcohol (e.g., red wine has many healthy properties and has been part of the Mediterranean-keto lifestyle for centuries).

The inability to tolerate saturated fats (as in they cause a lot of inflammation) might be genetic, and people with the APOE4 gene, which causes this inflammation, may also have an increased risk of heart disease and Alzheimer's disease.[37] Alcohol consumption also plays a part in the APOE4 gene. You see, heavy drinking has long been associated with increased risk of Alzheimer's disease, but people with the APOE4 gene have the same increased risk when they drink any alcohol![38]

Light drinkers and moderate drinkers who have the APOE4 gene should really not drink alcohol at all. Their genes think they are heavy drinkers, and the body responds accordingly.

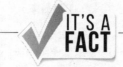

Drinking more than two alcoholic beverages a day isn't good for you, women especially. An occasional glass is fine but not daily. Use alcohol sparingly.

We all have APOE genes (E2, E3, and E4) from each of our parents, but only about 2 or 3 percent of us have both E4 genes. About 25 percent of people carry one copy of the APOE4 gene.[39] Patients with both copies of APOE4 gene have a 30–55 percent risk of developing mild cognitive impairment (MCI) or Alzheimer's disease by age eighty-five. Patients with only one copy of the E4 gene have a 20–25 percent risk of MCI or Alzheimer's disease.[40]

I have one E4 gene from one of my parents, and I've chosen to avoid alcohol almost completely. Very occasionally I will have red wine. It's simply not worth the increased risk of Alzheimer's disease.

If you have one or two APOE4 genes (you'll need to take a genotype test to find out), you should also be very mindful of alcohol consumption. If you happen to smoke and carry the APOE4 genes, you will really want to stop smoking! For APOE4 carriers, smoking creates elevated levels of oxidized LDL, which significantly increases the risk of heart disease.[41]

What helps you the most if you have one or two APOE4 genes? The answer: omega-3 (fish oil) with at least a 1:1 ratio or more of DHA to EPA. DHA is better for the brain. And now you know why I take four times what I recommend for everyone else.

On a keto diet, and the next-step Mediterranean-keto lifestyle, red wine is often recommended. In fact, red wine has proven health benefits but in moderation: one or two glasses with dinner, and less for women.[42]

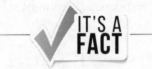

White wine has fewer benefits than red wine, and red wine is only healthy in moderation (one or two glasses per day or less), but if you have the APOE4 gene, you will probably want to avoid alcohol entirely.

For most patients on a healthy keto diet, I do not recommend red wine because it usually bumps them out of ketosis.

But to those who know they carry one or both APOE4 genes and those who have a strong family history of dementia, I recommend they avoid alcohol entirely or until they have their APOE gene test results. It's safer that way.

As for the very real benefits of red wine, those benefits can be found in other foods and supplements.[43] Either way, it's up to you. I personally take a red wine capsule daily that is high in the antioxidant resveratrol and polyphenols but contains no alcohol or carbs.

———

Those are the three biggest subtractions people on a keto diet should be applying to their lives. I would guess that very few keto dieters are aware of these subtractions, but they are vitally important.

Keep them out of your daily routine, for now and for the future. You will be glad you did!

Chapter 7

HOW YOU LOSE WEIGHT ON A KETO DIET

L OSING WEIGHT IS the number one reason people begin a keto diet. It only makes sense, because a keto diet revs up your metabolism rather than slowing it down. That alone is a great reason for choosing a keto diet to lose weight. But that is not all. Knowing how your body loses weight on a keto diet will help you in the weight loss process, and it will help you understand just how a keto diet prepares you to shift seamlessly into a Mediterranean-keto lifestyle.

The goal is to have a healthy lifestyle that you can enjoy while keeping the weight off. That is the end goal for every dieter. This is a win-win, and everyone likes that.

THE MACROS

When people say "macros," they are talking about the main food groups or macronutrients, such as carbs, proteins, and fats, that we consume on a daily basis. All food has these macros, just in different proportions.

The typical Western or American diet looks about like this:

- 50 percent carbs
- 34 percent fats
- 16 percent proteins[1]

On a pretty strict keto diet, where you are trying to lose weight or overcome a sickness or disease, it usually looks something like this:

- 75 percent fats
- 20 percent proteins

- 5 percent carbs

The more relaxed Mediterranean-keto lifestyle looks like this:

- 50–55 percent fats
- 20–25 percent proteins
- 20–25 percent carbs

You can easily see the differences. You can see where you might have been (the typical American diet), where you may need to go (a keto diet), and where you want to go after you have achieved a healthy weight (the Mediterranean-keto lifestyle).

The two biggest changes at the macro level between the typical American diet and a strict keto diet are the drastic decrease in carbs and the drastic increase in healthy fats.

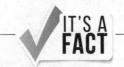

When carbs are reduced to below whatever your carb threshold is, you naturally start to lose weight.

For most people, dropping from a 50 percent carb daily intake to a mere 5 percent carb intake is in itself an effective weight loss program. But the increase in healthy fats, the decrease in carbs to only 5 percent, and the moderate protein intake of 20 percent are what turn the metabolism engines on, combat sickness and disease, and really get the diet kicked into high gear.

By healthy fats, I mean the fats that are found in such things as olive oil, avocado oil, nuts, seeds, omega-3 (fish oil), certain grass-fed meats, turkey, chicken, fish, some dairy, and more. We will discuss fats (and carbs and proteins) and how they work in the coming chapters.

HOW A KETO DIET WORKS

Our bodies typically burn sugar (glucose) for energy, and on a high-carb diet (45–65 percent, as is recommended by the US dietary guidelines), there is more than enough glucose to burn. Unfortunately any extra glucose is usually stored as fat, and the stored fat rarely burns off because the cells' energy factories (mitochondria) always burn glucose before they burn fat.

✔ IT'S A
FACT

Appetite control can be achieved only by breaking free of the carb cycle.

But there is plenty of glucose on hand, so the fat doesn't get a chance to be burned as fuel. And the cycle continues, year after year, pound after pound. In other words, the typical American high-carb diet is a weight-gaining and fat-gaining diet and never a fat-loss diet. It is simply almost impossible to burn fat for energy when sugars, carbs, and starches are consumed in excess. Because the body burns carbs preferentially (it is much easier and faster to metabolize a carb than a protein or fat), shifting the macros from a high-carb to a low-carb diet is the only way to break the cycle.

On a keto diet, you can't help but notice how different the macros are. And it's on purpose. You see, the low-carb, high-fat, moderate-protein diet eventually shifts your metabolism from burning sugars as fuel to burning fat as fuel.

Can protein be the energy source? Interestingly, the body turns excessive proteins into sugar, which is why a high-protein diet cannot work. If you eat too much protein, the body converts it to sugar, and you are back to where you started, only with protein as the source rather than carbs. Only a keto diet with its high-fat content can keep the body burning fat rather than reverting back to burning glucose for energy.

Technically what happens on a keto diet is that when your glucose levels, glycogen levels, and insulin levels get low enough, your body naturally shifts from burning sugar as fuel to burning fats and ketones as fuels, similar to a hybrid car that shifts from burning gasoline to using electric energy stored in batteries. During this ketosis process, because there is less glucose around, ketones and fats are burned as energy.

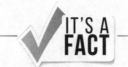

Approximately 84 percent of the ketones that are produced in the body are oxidized (burned as fuel), and the rest are excreted in the urine or exhaled.[2]

Ketones are produced in the liver from the body breaking down fats to produce energy, and this is called fat oxidation. That means that your body is burning fat. That is a metabolism on fire!

Exercise usually isn't even required for this fat burning to begin, but adding light exercise (such as walking twenty to thirty minutes three to five times a week) will help speed up the process. And that is the power and effectiveness of a keto diet.

These ketones and fats are used to produce energy, and then some are exhaled or flushed out of your body through your urine, which is why you can measure these small amounts of ketones with a blood ketone meter, a ketone breath meter, or a urine ketone test strip. On a urine ketone test strip, you can look at the color of the urine strip and tell if you are in ketosis. The strips are convenient and very easy to use.

For the first month or two on a keto diet, these simple, easy, inexpensive urine test strips are handy and help you know if you are in ketosis and burning fat rather than still burning sugar as fuel. When your body is accustomed to ketosis and burning fats for fuel, the urine ketone test strips lose some of their accuracy. A small pinprick on the finger to test your blood or a breath meter are more effective methods at that point. These blood ketone meters aren't that expensive, but the blood ketone test strips themselves are usually a few dollars each test. Nutritional ketosis is 0.5 to 1.0 millimoles and optimal ketosis is 1.5 to 3.0 millimoles on the blood meter.[3]

Most people will soon get a feel for being in ketosis, but for my patients who are battling obesity, sickness, or disease, especially cancer, I do recommend testing for ketones for at least the first three to six months on a keto diet. But it's entirely up to you.

HOW A NORMAL DIET DOES *NOT* WORK

When averaged out, the typical American diet is 50 percent carbs, 34 percent fats, and 16 percent proteins. With this as the foundation, the results are going to continue to be the same: fat gaining and rarely ever fat burning. Always and forever, it cannot be anything but this because of how the body works.

That alone is bad news, but here is where things get worse. When you eat carbs, your body produces more insulin to handle the blood-sugar spikes. These energy fluctuations naturally happen throughout the day as you eat. But what's interesting is that the higher insulin level is instructing your body to store those carb calories as fat.[4] And not only does the insulin prompt the storage of fat; it also blocks the release of fat that is stored as fat in the body.[5] In other words, insulin programs your body to store fat, then locks it away!

Also, as we have discussed, these insulin spikes throughout the day eventually lead to insulin resistance, inflammation, and a host of sicknesses and diseases. And with increased insulin resistance, more insulin is produced to try to remove the excess sugar from the blood, and all the while the insulin is telling your body to store even more fat. Is it any wonder why obesity leads directly to prediabetes and type 2 diabetes? That's simply the body doing its thing.

A keto diet, on the other hand, drastically reduces insulin production. After all, if there are no sugar spikes, there is no need for your body to produce excess insulin to lower the blood sugar. Insulin levels drop and inflammation fades. And your body's constant instructions to store fat are silenced.

For example, the following food choices basically show a few of the food options on a typical American diet versus a keto diet:

- 1 cup pasta (41 grams carbs) or 1 cup zucchini noodles (3 grams carbs)

- 1 cup rice (44 grams carbs) or 1 cup shirataki rice (0 grams carbs)

- 1 cup mashed potatoes (44 grams carbs) or 1 cup mashed cauliflower (8 grams carbs)

- 4 ounces french fries (44 grams carbs) or zucchini fries in air fryer (3 grams carbs)

- 3.5 ounces potato chips (46 grams carbs) or 1 ounce mixed nuts (4 grams carbs)[6]

The cup of pasta, for example, with its 41 grams of carbs, is going to cause an insulin spike as the body tries to lower the blood sugar. On the other hand, the cup of zucchini noodles, with its 3 grams of healthy carbs, would hardly cause a blip on the insulin radar.

CONTROLLING YOUR APPETITE

For many, appetite control is the coveted control switch. It's the holy grail. They know that if they can control their appetite, they can control their food intake and their weight.

But on a typical weight loss program, if you manage to lose weight, your metabolism slows down and your body thinks it's starving. So as an act of self-preservation, the hunger hormone ghrelin is released to make you hungry so you will eat. And leptin, the hormone that tells you when you are full, slows down. This combined duo of self-sabotage is precisely why as many as 95 percent of people who lose weight on a typical diet regain it all, and often more, within five years.[7]

The surest way to have a ravenous appetite is to eat a lot of carbs (carbohydrates, sugars, or starches). It's a roller coaster that never stops going, for whenever you run low on glucose (about three to four hours after you eat), your ghrelin hormone cranks back up and you eat more carbs, which sends the roller coaster up, only to come back down again. Up and down, around and around, there is no pause or exit.

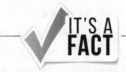

IT'S A FACT

Intermittent fasting is when you feed your body only one or two meals a day in an eight-hour window and you fast for the other sixteen hours. Eating a late breakfast and an early dinner is one way to do this. Intermittent fasting helps your body enter ketosis faster and burn fat as fuel.

But it's different on a keto diet. The high-fat intake on a keto diet is what makes you feel full, satiated, and satisfied. And because fat takes a long time to digest, it releases energy slowly, so your body doesn't think it's starving. That is how the ghrelin and leptin hormones don't sabotage you when you are on a keto diet.[8]

Fiber also plays an important role in curbing your appetite. The recommended 2 tablespoons of psyllium husk powder does wonders to make you feel full, not to mention the countless other health benefits that come from adequate fiber intake. In fact, both fat and fiber help suppress your hunger by lowering your levels of ghrelin, which is the principal feed-me-now appetite hormone.

So it is possible! You can control your appetite hormones on a keto diet. And then when you shift over to the Mediterranean-keto lifestyle, which is also low-carb, high fat, and moderate protein, your appetite hormones will remain under your control forever!

WHAT TO DO WHEN YOUR WEIGHT LOSS PLATEAUS

Everyone hits a plateau when they are trying to lose weight. This is true, even on a keto diet. I've found that about 90 percent of the people who go on a keto diet do so to lose weight, and 100 percent of them hit weight loss plateaus along the way. Every single one of my patients who has gone on a keto diet has hit a plateau.

The way to think of weight loss is to see it as a flight of stairs. You lose weight; then it slows or stops for a few weeks, so you wait or adjust something, and weight usually drops again; then it slows or stops, so you can wait or adjust again, and on and on. You are simply stairstepping and making a series of adjustments. That is all. Nothing is wrong with you. You may have simply maxed out or slowed your weight loss with what you are doing. The answer is to either continue on the keto diet or make a minor adjustment to break through a plateau.

One of my patients started on a keto diet. She lost weight from retained water and belly fat first. She was happy, losing about one pound per week. Then, after about two months, she plateaued. She was eating a little too much food (at the macro level), so we dialed back her overall caloric intake from 2,200 calories a day to 1,800 calories a day. She started losing weight again, around one pound per week, for several months. Then she plateaued again.

We decreased her caloric intake to 1,600 calories a day, and she started losing weight again. Then she plateaued again. This time, we looked at her exercise regimen and added walking to her routine. For her, it was a twenty-minute walk three times per week. She started losing weight again, about half a pound to one pound a week. This continued for several months. And yet again she plateaued.

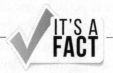

To lose one pound of fat, you need to burn 3,500 calories.

We then decreased her meals from three a day to two a day, with a keto coffee in the morning. In her coffee she used one scoop of MCT oil powder instead of the coffee creamer with sucralose that she had been using. (Sucralose is an obesogen.) She started losing weight again.

This happened several more times. Once we needed to increase her fats (increasing the amount of olive oil per meal). One time she was eating too many nuts. Another time we checked her thyroid, which turned out to be sluggish (she had cold feet and hands, was losing her outer eyebrows, and had dry skin), and I put her on a natural thyroid supplement. Then a big life event happened that caused a lot of stress, and she stopped losing weight. She rested, took some hemp oil drops to help calm her nerves, and focused on getting a good night's sleep. Within a few weeks she started losing weight again. Eventually she reached a weight she liked. For her, that was the end of the stairs. She was happy.

I have had hundreds of patients just like this. Sure, each person's situation is unique, but there are usually only a limited number of reasons weight plateaus.

If you are over age sixty (especially for women), keep in mind that it does take a little longer to lose weight and your plateaus will usually last longer. Stick with it, for it will work, just a little more slowly.

NET CARBS

Total Carbs – Fiber = Net Carbs

Example: a small handful of almonds has 6 grams of carbs – 3.5 grams of fiber = 2.5 grams of net carbs

And if you do cheat, that's OK. It's not the end of the world. It will simply slow down your weight loss efforts. So if you cheat, forgive yourself and move on. Press on.

Speaking of averages, the average adult woman in the United States consumes around 1,600–2,400 calories in food per day. To lose weight, women should decrease their food intake to 1,600–2,000 calories per day while maintaining the macros of 75 percent fats, 5 percent carbs, and 20 percent proteins.

For adult men, their average is 2,400–3,800 calories per day. To lose weight, men should decrease their food intake to 2,000–2,400 calories per day while maintaining the macros of 75 percent fats, 5 percent carbs, and 20 percent proteins.

When you hit a plateau, the question to ask yourself is, "What is causing this?" Then you look at all the facts on the table. And let me say that it's not a real stall or plateau until you have been there for three to four weeks. Don't pressure yourself. You don't have to lose weight every single week. After three to four full weeks have gone by, you can call it a stall. Following are several things to consider if you hit a plateau. Use and reuse this list each time you find yourself at a plateau:

- Am I eating too many carbs? Even healthy carbs count. At the macro level, 5 percent of your daily intake coming from healthy carbs should be enough to burn fat for most anyone. That's 20 grams of healthy net carbs per day. Odds are your carb intake has crept up and is greater than 5 percent (20 grams).

- Am I eating too much protein? If you eat an excessive amount of protein, the body will convert the excess protein to carbs, and that can throw you out of ketosis. Usually 3–4 ounces of protein per meal for women and 3–6 ounces of protein per meal for men is adequate. Some people need less.

- Am I drinking enough water? Not drinking enough water can slow weight loss down. Increase your water intake to at least six to eight glasses per day.

- Am I eating too many nuts? Eating too many nuts, which may have excessive net carbs, can knock you out of ketosis. Or maybe the excessive proteins from too many nuts are converting to sugar, which definitely would stop ketosis and weight loss.

- Do I need to start exercising? You may need to add brisk walking to your routine. Start with ten to twenty minutes of walking, three times each week. You want to eventually increase it to thirty minutes or more five days a week, but for now this is a good start. But just walk; don't run. Also, if you are able, find a walking partner for accountability.

- Am I eating too much dairy? Dairy is often the culprit for slowing down and even stalling weight loss. Look at what you've been eating. Adjust if necessary.

- Am I eating enough fat? Double-check your 75 percent fats intake. Are you still on target? Adding more olive oil, avocado oil, almond oil, or macadamia nut oil to meals is often the answer. For women, 75 percent of 1,600 total calories as fat is 10 tablespoons per day (3.33 tablespoons per meal). For men, 75 percent of 2,400 total calories as fat is 15 tablespoons per day (5 table-spoons per meal).

- Am I consuming too much food (calories)? Maybe you are simply eating too much food. Look at your daily intake. Are you on target (1,600 calories per day for women and 2,000–2,400 calories per day for men)? Count your calories for a few days to check yourself.

- Am I consuming artificial sweeteners? Fake sugars are notorious for knocking you out of ketosis. Examine your food and drinks closely.

- Are there hidden sugars in my diet? Examine your food and drinks. Nut butters, for example, which are great for fat and protein intake, often have sugar added and may even have excessive carbs.

- Do I need to increase my exercise? If you want to increase your exercise (beyond the assumed twenty-minute walks three times a week), increase your walks to thirty minutes four or five times a week. Do more aerobic exercise, ride a bike, swim, or find some other activity you enjoy.

- Do I need to begin intermittent fasting? On a keto diet you will feel full longer and can usually skip meals, especially breakfasts. This increases your fat burning. Maintain your macros as you go. Many of my female patients are able to break through their weight loss plateaus by eating their last meals between 5:00 and 6:00 p.m.

- Am I under stress? Stress releases cortisol, which can cause weight gain. Stress may be unavoidable, so learn to practice techniques that calm you. Meditation, praise music, prayer, laughter, sleep, reading books (especially the Bible), watching funny movies or TV shows, drinking tea, turning off technology, using essential oils, playing with your grandkids, or journaling are all good ways to decrease stress. If you are able to fix the situation and remove the stressor, that is always the best option. (My book *Stress Less* is a good resource if you need to break free from stress in your life.)

- Are my hormones fluctuating? Women have hormone fluctuations during their menstrual cycles, especially during their menstrual periods, and this can slow down weight loss (typically for a week). If this happens, be aware, but press on.

- Am I getting enough sleep? Getting a good night's sleep, seven to eight hours, is vital. Some people need less sleep, but odds are you need to regularly get at least seven to eight hours each night.

- Is my thyroid sluggish? Consult your doctor for this, or read my book *Dr. Colbert's Hormone Health Zone*, but a sluggish thyroid is common (especially in women) as we age. Symptoms often include cold hands and feet, losing the outer eyebrows, a lower body temperature, constant fatigue, weight gain, constipation, and dry skin. A natural thyroid supplement is usually the answer here. (See appendix A, "Recommended Supplements.")

- Am I consuming too much sodium? Too much salt can slow down your weight loss. I've seen it happen. Look closely at your food intake. You may need to cut back on the salt and salty seasonings you might be using.

- Am I getting too much exercise? If you do high-intensity exercise, your body has to burn glucose for energy (protein and fat burn too slowly), so you will need to increase your carbs before a workout. (Or take MCT oil powder or Instant Ketones before a workout.) Otherwise, your body will crash, you may need to sleep, and you may feel sick. All you need to do is increase your carbs before or on those high-intensity-workout days. Eventually you will find the balance. It's best to avoid high-intensity workouts until you achieve your weight loss goals, or you will probably have to increase your carbs before your workouts.

Remember, weight loss is like a flight of stairs. You will drop, plateau, drop, plateau, and so on. A plateau is never a sign that you can't lose weight or that a keto diet doesn't work. Don't panic. Honestly evaluate where you are and what you are doing, and adjust. And keep going. Eventually and inevitably you will reach a weight that you like. It's a weight that gives you the health and freedom you want.

And that is the time when I recommend you shift over to the Mediterranean-keto lifestyle. As you live the Mediterranean-keto lifestyle, you will drift in and out of ketosis (as before a hard workout when you increase your carbs somewhat). This lifestyle will give you continued health, flexibility, and freedom. That is where you want to be.

That's where we all want to be!

Chapter 8

UNDERSTANDING FATS (MACRO 1)

A T ITS CORE, what makes a keto diet work is the fact that your body can burn fat continuously as a healthy, clean, efficient source of fuel. That is the core macro of a keto diet. If you are trying to get into the metabolic state of ketosis and burn fat so you lose weight (or fight sickness or disease), that means your daily fat intake on a keto diet is going to be up around 70–75 percent of your daily calories, with the addition of a moderate protein and a very low carb intake.

For many of us, that is scary, daunting, and illogical. We don't want to get fat, yet we are told to eat fats, and by eating more fat, we burn more fat and store less fat. How is that even possible?

Understanding fats is vital to your health, whether you are eating the typical American cuisine, losing weight on a keto diet, or living the Mediterranean-keto lifestyle. It pays to know what you are putting in your mouth and why.

THE FOUR FAT OPTIONS

Spend a few minutes researching fats, and you will quickly discover that there are four very different types of fat that come into play with the foods we eat. Here they are:

1. Monounsaturated fatty acids (MUFAs)—These fats are good for you, are good for your heart, lower bad cholesterol, raise good cholesterol, lower heart attack and stroke risk, improve insulin sensitivity, make you feel full, and help you lose weight. They are found in olive oil, avocado oil, nut oils, seeds, nuts, nut butters, and

so on. Canola oil is high in monounsaturated fats, but most is genetically modified, and I don't recommend it.

2. Saturated fatty acids (SFAs)—These fats are good in low amounts and sometimes in moderation but not good for you when eaten with excessive carbs or sugars or eaten in excess. They are found in fatty meats, cheese, cream, butter, ghee, coconut oil, sour cream, ice cream, whipped cream, MCT oil, palm oil, and palm kernel oil.

3. Polyunsaturated fatty acids (PUFAs)—Some of these fats are very good, and some are very bad. The good ones are found in omega-3 fats in a natural form, while the bad ones are usually in a processed form. Frying with polyunsaturated fats causes overproduction of reactive oxygen species (ROS) such as hydrogen peroxide, superoxide, and hydroxyl, which are free radicals that can damage antioxidant defense systems, causing oxidative stress. They can eventually lead to heart disease, cancers, and neurodegenerative diseases.[1] Restaurants usually deep-fry french fries in vegetable oils, including peanut oil, corn oil, canola oil, or sunflower oil. Good PUFAs are found in salmon, mackerel, sardines, flaxseeds, chia seeds, hemp seeds, walnuts, and more. Bad PUFAs are found in corn oil, sunflower oil, cottonseed oil, soybean oil, safflower oil, most vegetable oils, and so on, which are omega-6 polyunsaturated fats. Good omega-6 fats include pecans, almonds, cashews, macadamia nuts, pistachios, pine nuts, and hazelnuts. You should never eat food fried in polyunsaturated fats.

4. Trans fats—These fats are simply bad. They are chemically created (look for *hydrogenated, partially hydrogenated,* or *shortening* on the label), are cheap to make, and have a long shelf life. They are also very bad news

for your heart, brain, cholesterol levels, weight loss plans, and more. They are found in restaurants and many packaged foods. Foods high in trans fats include stick margarine, many nondairy creamers, cakes (especially the icing), cookies, pies, shortening, microwave popcorn, and frozen pizza.[2]

When you're on a keto diet, and really for anyone who wants to be healthy, the fats you want to be eating are the good ones. That includes the monounsaturated fats, limited amounts of saturated fats, and the good polyunsaturated fats. Conversely, the fats to avoid are the bad polyunsaturated fats, trans fats, and foods fried in polyunsaturated fats. (Most often those are high-carb foods, such as potato chips and french fries.)

But it's easier said than done! Most people, especially if they are starting on a keto diet, are surprised at just how hard it is to avoid bad fats. They seem to be everywhere. On a keto diet you wouldn't be eating things such as cookies, donuts, fried chicken, and frozen pizza anyway, but the point is, trans fats and bad polyunsaturated fats are often hidden where you would not expect them. When it comes down to it, your job is to make sure you only consume the good fats and avoid the bad. That's all there is to it.

PUT GOOD FATS TO WORK FOR YOU

Fat is a tool that you can actually use to your advantage. That seems strange to say, but it's true. For example, you already know that fat helps control the hunger hormone (ghrelin), so when you eat fats or add more fats (e.g., olive oil) to your food, you are purposefully using fats to keep those hunger cravings in check. And that helps you lose weight.

You know that the right fats are a healthy, efficient source of energy for your body, so maintaining a high-fat diet (75 percent on a keto diet, then 50 percent when you shift over to the Mediterranean-keto lifestyle) will keep your metabolism running.

But did you know that you can use fat to fight the number one killer in America, cardiovascular disease? In one large study (called the Lyon Diet Heart Study), they took seven thousand people already at risk of heart attack and death and had them eat a Mediterranean-style diet full of olive oil and omega-3 (fish oil). Their risk of heart attack and death dropped by 30 percent![3]

NET CARBS

Good fats to eat:

- extra-virgin olive oil
- avocado oil
- walnut oil
- almond oil
- macadamia oil
- unrefined sesame oil
- tahini
- flax oil
- hemp oil
- avocados, olives, and other plants
- nuts and seeds

Fats that are OK to eat in small amounts, about 10 percent of fat intake (about 1 tablespoon for women and 1 1/2–2 tablespoons for men):

- butter from grass-fed, pastured cows or goats
- grass-fed ghee
- organic, humanely raised lard, tallow, duck fat, or chicken fat
- coconut oil
- MCT oil
- sustainable palm oil

Fats to avoid:

- soybean oil
- canola oil
- corn oil
- safflower oil
- sunflower oil
- peanut oil
- vegetable oil
- grapeseed oil
- vegetable shortening
- margarine
- butter substitutes
- anything that is hydrogenated[4]

Or maybe you are considering taking statin drugs (despite the side effects). That same seven-thousand-person Lyon Diet Heart Study found that the decreased risk of heart attack and death was equal to what statin drugs would have offered.[5]

In another study, they were even able to quantify the fat intake and connect it to an actual percentage of health improvement. Specifically they found that increasing olive oil consumption by 10 grams per day reduced the risk of cardiovascular disease and death risk by 10 percent and 7 percent, respectively.[6] That is only 0.75 tablespoons of olive oil per day. That's pretty easy to do and highly motivating with that type of return.

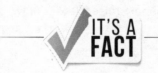

Healthy fat sources: cold-pressed avocado oil, cold-pressed macadamia oil, cold-pressed almond oil, extra-virgin olive oil, olives, walnuts, and avocados

Perhaps the biggest motivation for all of us to eat more healthy fats should be how it benefits the brain. Olive oil specifically is great fuel for the brain. The entire keto diet is excellent for the brain, but it's the good fats (olive oil, in particular) that feed the brain and make it happy. Omega-3 (fish oil), nut oils, and avocado oil are also excellent oils for the brain.

If you've wondered why brain fog usually disappears soon after starting a keto diet, it's usually because of the good anti-inflammatory fats, especially fish oil and olive oil. The brain thrives on them, as opposed to sugars, carbs, and starches. And there are the proven benefits of a keto diet in fighting memory-related diseases such as dementia and Alzheimer's. It's the good fats that fight on your behalf.

Another reason to eat good fats is the fact that fats help your body absorb the fat-soluble vitamins that are in plants. Without the right fats, even eating the right plants is less healthy for you.

Lastly, eating more of the right fats has been found to decrease the risk of stroke, cancer, heart disease, type 2 diabetes, and obesity.[7] These are not bad reasons for purposefully adding healthy fats to your diet, now, are they?

AVOID BAD FATS TO YOUR BENEFIT

Just as good fats help your body tremendously, so bad fats can do a lot of damage to your heart, brain, arteries, gut, energy levels, and waistline.

You already know what the bad fats are:

- trans fats
- some polyunsaturated fats (e.g., oils such as soy, corn, cottonseed, etc.)
- canola oil, a GMO monounsaturated fat
- excessive saturated fats (e.g., cheese, butter, etc.), especially if eaten with carbs or sugars or without sufficient omega-3 fats in your body

And you've seen some of the damage these fats help cause in our bodies, such as

- insulin resistance
- inflammation
- heart attacks
- stroke
- type 2 diabetes
- leaky gut
- increased bad cholesterol
- decreased good cholesterol
- dementia
- Alzheimer's disease.

For example, trans fats (among other things) increase the risk of heart attack, heart disease, stroke, and type 2 diabetes; raise bad, LDL cholesterol; increase triglyceride levels (which hardens the arteries); and lower good, HDL cholesterol.[8] That in itself is a lot of damage.

Polyunsaturated fats have been found to raise your blood pressure, increase your risk of blood clots that can cause heart attacks and strokes, and cause an increase in inflammatory diseases, such as cardiovascular disease, obesity, and Alzheimer's disease.[9] They also slow metabolism, increase estrogen levels, create hormonal imbalances, suppress the immune system, accelerate aging, and more.[10] These polyunsaturated fats also oxidize quickly, especially from repeated use or sunlight. These fats have been linked to increased cancer risk.[11]

IT'S A FACT

Sunshine will denature olive oil. Optimally, buy olive oil in dark glass containers, and always store in a dark pantry.

And with saturated fats, as we have already discussed, they cause inflammation when eaten with refined carbs or sugar or when you don't have enough omega-3 in your system. But people should worry more about the effect of sugar and starch on their cholesterol levels than the effect of saturated fat in grass-fed beef.[12] Part of the problem is that we typically overeat saturated fats, especially in the form of dairy and meat. We really only need 7–10 percent saturated fats in our daily diet. So if you keep your saturated fat intake to less than 10 percent, you are doing well.

But knowing the increased risks, the symptoms, and the diseases is seldom sufficient motivation for change. After all, we have known of the dangers of these fats for decades, but restaurants don't change, factories still produce packaged foods with these fats, the FDA allows them, and the USDA recommends many of them. If you eat out at restaurants a lot, chances are you are consuming a lot of these cheap, inflammatory fats, especially if you eat at fast food restaurants. The only option is really the first and best option: you choosing what you put in your mouth.

When you start on a keto diet, one of the first steps is to go through your pantry and get rid of (or donate to charity) the foods that don't fit your new keto diet and your eventual Mediterranean-keto lifestyle.

WHEN COOKING WITH FATS

Every fat you might use to cook has a temperature at which it starts to smoke and then burn. This temperature is the smoke point, where the fat oxidizes. As you know, oxidized fat causes inflammation and free radicals, so you naturally want to cook without oxidizing the fat.

For example, the smoke point of extra-virgin olive oil is just 160°C/320°F, while the smoke point of avocado oil is 271°C/570°F. Both of these are healthy fats, but if you are frying an egg, use avocado oil. If you are drizzling these oils over your green salad, you can use either or both. Because each fat has its own smoke point, each fat has a recommended use. Consider the following:

- flaxseed oil—smoke point: 107°C/225°F—drizzle, dressing

- extra-virgin olive oil—smoke point: 160°C/320°F— drizzle, sauté

- butter—smoke point: 177°C/350°F—drizzle, sauté (limited amounts)

- coconut oil—smoke point: 177°C/350°F—drizzle, sauté (limited amounts)

- macadamia nut oil—smoke point: 199°C/390°F

- almond oil—smoke point: 216°C/420°F

- ghee—smoke point: 252°C/485°F—sear, stir-fry (limited amounts)

- avocado oil—smoke point: 271°C/570°F—sear, stir-fry[13]

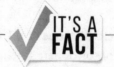

IT'S A FACT

Start low and go slow on olive oil and MCT oil. I usually encourage patients to start with just 1 tablespoon of olive oil on their salad or food to avoid loose stools and then gradually increase the amount. MCT oil can also cause loose stools, but the other oils, including avocado and nut oils and nut butters, rarely cause diarrhea.

Making a change to your daily routine like using the correct healthy fat is easy enough. It's knowing what is good and what is most healthy that makes all the difference. If you break fats into one group for cooking and one for adding to raw or cooked foods, it would look something like this:

- For cooking: avocado oil, almond oil, macadamia nut oil (or palm kernel oil, ghee, or coconut oil, all in small amounts)

- For putting on your raw or already-cooked food: olive oil, avocado oil, walnut oil, flaxseed oil, hazelnut oil, almond oil, macadamia nut oil, cocoa butter, avocados, guacamole, and saturated fats, including full-fat coconut milk, grass-fed butter, grass-fed ghee, MCT oil, coconut oil, coconut meat, coconut cream, unsweetened coconut milk yogurt, and unsweetened almond milk yogurt, in limited amounts[14]

On a keto diet you will get most of your healthy fats from the fats that you add to your raw or already-cooked foods. Nuts, seeds, fish, and omega-3 supplements are also important sources of healthy fats.

Now that you better understand fats, you are more prepared for healthy living!

Chapter 9

UNDERSTANDING PROTEINS (MACRO 2)

THE SECOND CORE macro of a keto diet is the moderate intake of healthy proteins. In addition to healthy fats, your body requires healthy proteins to live and function properly.

Protein comes from many sources, and each source is unique. Some protein sources have vitamins and minerals that your body needs, while some protein sources come with built-in carbs that will bump you out of ketosis if you eat too much. Some proteins are more suited for when you shift over to the Mediterranean-keto lifestyle, and some proteins are hard to come by or are expensive, which means a supplement is the best option in those cases.

Remember, if you eat too much protein, your body will start to convert the excess protein into glucose, and you are back to burning sugar as your body's fuel source. This of course stops a keto diet from working.

The amount you want to aim for while on your keto diet is about 1 gram of protein per 2.2 pounds (1 kilogram) of your body's weight per day. Calculating that per day and per meal, it would look something like this:

- 125-pound person: 57 grams per day, or 19 grams proteins per meal (about 3 ounces)

- 150-pound person: 68 grams per day, or 23 grams proteins per meal (about 3.5 ounces)

- 180-pound person: 82 grams per day, or 27 grams proteins per meal (about 4 ounces)

- 250-pound person: 114 grams per day, or 38 grams proteins per meal (about 5.5 ounces)

Keep in mind that women usually need less protein per day than men (about one-third to one-half less).

On a keto diet, with the usual goal of weight loss or with doctor's orders getting well again, keeping your protein intake in range is vital.

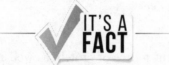

Pasture-raised poultry and eggs are best; these birds freely roam around and eat their natural diet. The next best is organic. That at least guarantees it's not full of antibiotics or fed grains sprayed with pesticides.[1]

HEALTHY PROTEINS

Each ounce of protein (e.g., egg, chicken, cheese, fish, turkey, steak, beans) on average has about 7 grams of protein in it. But as you well know, not all proteins are created equal.

Here are several healthy protein sources:

Eggs

Eggs are a superfood. They include all the amino acids that we need, all in one source. The egg yolk "is the most nutritious part—low in calories, high in protein, and full of vitamins, minerals, antioxidants, choline, and phytonutrients."[2]

People are more commonly allergic to the whites than the yellow yolk. If you are sensitive to either, simply rotate or use in the way that causes no problems.

The best eggs are pasture-raised eggs, which studies have shown contain two and a half times as many omega-3 fats.[3] Pasture-raised eggs can include chicken, duck, goose, ostrich, or quail.[4]

Meat

Meat in moderation, keeping to your intake per meal per day, is a good source of protein. Grass-fed meat is higher in vitamins and antioxidants than grain-fed meat.[5] If you use grass-fed meat, then you don't have to do leaner cuts, but if you don't use grass-fed meat, then choose leaner cuts (which have fewer toxins). The best sources of protein from meat include grass-fed beef, buffalo, goat, lamb, and pork; pasture-raised chicken, duck, pheasant, quail, and turkey; and wild boar, elk, rabbit, and deer.[6]

Fish

Fish are an excellent source of protein as well as necessary omega-3 (fish oil). However, for the amount of omega-3 we need per day, using supplements is a realistic option for most people.

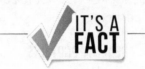

7 grams of protein = 1 ounce (e.g., 4 ounces of fish = 28 grams of protein)

Also, not all fish are equal. Smaller fish are less likely to have mercury, and farmed-raised fish typically have more omega-6 and less omega-3 fats from the foods they are fed, and more toxins and less protein per pound. I simply recommend eating as much wild fish as you can. One excellent reason: diets rich with wild-caught fish are associated with a 60 percent decrease in Alzheimer's.[7] The best fish to eat are wild caught or sustainably harvested, farm-raised salmon, mackerel, herring, anchovies, and sardines.[8]

Beans

Beans are a good source of protein and fiber, but they are best to avoid or to eat in small amounts (such as one-quarter to one-half cup) of low-starch beans (lentils, lupini, snow peas, black-eyed peas, mung beans, etc.) when on a keto diet. Later you can eat more varieties of beans and in larger amounts as part of your Mediterranean-keto lifestyle.

Why wait? A single cup of cooked pinto beans, for example, which would provide you with 12 grams of protein, would also include 35 grams of carbs! That's more than enough to stall your keto diet for the day. A small, 2-ounce piece of salmon, on the other hand, would get you the same amount of protein but with no carbs.[9]

The seldom-mentioned lupini bean is high in both protein and fiber yet has very few net carbs. The starch is indigestible in your gut, so it does not make your blood-sugar levels go up and is an acceptable bean for a keto diet.[10] Until you shift to the Mediterranean-keto lifestyle, it's best to avoid higher-starch beans (such as peas, lima beans, kidney beans, baked beans, pintos, etc.).

With your dried beans, soak them overnight in water with a little salt, and discard the water the next morning, then pressure-cook for at least seven and a half minutes. This soaking and cooking will help remove the lectins and decrease inflammation and gas.

If you happen to have gut dysbiosis or an autoimmune disease or are obese or diabetic, then you should eliminate beans from your diet until your gut is healthy.[11] Then you can add them in slowly and always in small amounts as long as they are soaked and then pressure-cooked for at least seven and a half minutes.

Dairy

Dairy (cheese, cream, yogurt, cottage cheese, cream cheese, etc.) is a great source of protein, but with it (as we have discussed) come a lot of saturated fats and PCBs (toxins). If you choose to eat dairy while on your keto diet, I recommend small amounts.

As for cheese, goat and sheep cheeses, like feta, are lower in saturated fats, have fewer carbs, and are less likely to cause inflammation. (One of the most common food sensitivities is dairy.[12]) If you do eat cheese, use it in small amounts on your salads as a garnish.

Soy

What about soy? It has been touted as a great source of protein, but I do not recommend soy protein or soybean oil. In fact, the soy protein in fake meats, bars, and shakes is chemically altered and is a byproduct of the soybean oil production process, but non-GMO, organic, traditional soybean foods like tofu, tempeh, miso, natto, and gluten-free soy sauce or tamari would be fine.[13]

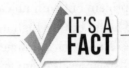

Look for

- pasture-raised poultry and eggs
- wild or sustainably harvested fish, shrimp, oysters, etc.
- grass-fed beef, bison, pork, sheep, goat, etc.
- wild deer, rabbit, elk, etc.
- organic or non-GMO nuts, beans, seeds, etc.

Nuts

Nuts are a great source of protein, as well as fat, fiber, vitamins, and minerals, and they are readily available, relatively inexpensive, and usually toxin-free. They have been found to help prevent many chronic diseases (cancer, diabetes, neurodegenerative diseases, cardio-vascular diseases, diabetes, etc.) and reduce blood pressure and cho-lesterol levels.[14]

Here are several common nuts and their related breakdowns that will help you on your keto diet. The information is based on a 1-ounce serving (a small handful, or about 28 grams).[15]

- Almonds
  * Calories: 161
  * Fat: 14 grams
  * Protein: 6 grams
  * Carbs: 6 grams
  * Fiber: 3.5 grams
  * Total net carbs: 2.5 grams (very keto-friendly nut)

- Pistachios

  * Calories: 156
  * Fat: 12.5 grams
  * Protein: 6 grams
  * Carbs: 8 grams
  * Fiber: 3 grams
  * Total net carbs: 5 grams

- Walnuts

  * Calories: 182
  * Fat: 18 grams
  * Protein: 4 grams
  * Carbs: 4 grams
  * Fiber: 2 grams
  * Total net carbs: 2 grams (very keto-friendly nut)

- Cashews

  * Calories: 155
  * Fat: 12 grams
  * Protein: 5 grams
  * Carbs: 9 grams
  * Fiber: 1 grams
  * Total net carbs: 8 grams (Caution: this is a higher-carb nut.)

- Pecans

  * Calories: 193
  * Fat: 20 grams
  * Protein: 3 grams

* Carbs: 4 grams
* Fiber: 2.5 grams
* Total net carbs: 1.5 grams (very keto-friendly nut)

- Macadamia nuts

  * Calories: 200
  * Fat: 21 grams
  * Protein: 2 grams
  * Carbs: 4 grams
  * Fiber: 2.5 grams
  * Total net carbs: 1.5 grams (very keto-friendly nut)

- Brazil nuts

  * Calories: 182
  * Fat: 18 grams
  * Protein: 4 grams
  * Carbs: 3 grams
  * Fiber: 2 grams
  * Total net carbs: 1 gram (Caution: Brazil nuts are very high in selenium, and just a single nut has 68–91 micrograms of selenium. The recommended adult allowance is 55 micrograms.[16])

- Hazelnuts

  * Calories: 176
  * Fat: 9 grams
  * Protein: 6 grams
  * Carbs: 6 grams
  * Fiber: 3.5 grams
  * Total net carbs: 2.5 grams

- Peanuts (Peanuts are not a tree nut but rather a legume. They do, however, have similar health benefits.)

  * Calories: 176
  * Fat: 17 grams
  * Protein: 4 grams
  * Carbs: 5 grams
  * Fiber: 3 grams
  * Total net carbs: 2 grams

Believe it or not, many packaged nuts are often sprayed with inflammatory oils, such as soy or canola oil, so read the labels carefully.[17] One answer to this problem is to buy nuts or seeds in their raw form, then soak them overnight (to remove lectins and phytates, which often cause inflammation) before lightly roasting them in the oven (or you can use a dehydrator). Season to taste.

Thankfully there are many different proteins to choose from. And when you shift from your keto diet to the Mediterranean-keto lifestyle, you will have even more proteins to choose from.

Perfection is not required, so relax. There is no perfect plan for eating the exactly right protein. Simply do your best, and work toward your health goals.

Now that you better understand proteins, you are more prepared for healthy living!

Chapter 10

UNDERSTANDING CARBS (MACRO 3)

T
HE THIRD AND final core macro of a keto diet is the low intake of healthy carbs. Technically, for your body to function properly at the cellular level, you need only fat and protein, not carbohydrates. What that means is that the low-carb keto diet certainly won't kill you!

Carbs are everywhere and in almost everything we eat. On a keto diet there are two foundational principles regarding carbs:

1. Keep your daily carb count really low (20 grams of net carbs).

2. Make those carbs count by eating healthy carbs.

The low-carb side of a keto diet is what forces your body into fat-burning mode. It is the primary reason for weight loss or for preventing or treating a sickness or disease.

Over the years, I have found that the number one reason my patients' weight loss plateaus, the number one reason they get bumped out of the fat-burning mode of ketosis, and the number one reason for weight gain is simply eating too many carbs. In other words, as much as you may enjoy carbs in their various forms, they are what stand between you and your health goals. So don't let carbs, which your body technically does not need, get in your way.

YOUR DAILY CARB GOAL

On a keto diet, your goal is to limit your carbs to about 5 percent of your total daily intake. That low number is almost always low enough to burn fat for everyone, regardless of gender, age, or physical condition.

With carbs that low, the body eventually shifts from burning sugar for fuel to burning fat for fuel.

That 5 percent of daily intake usually translates into about 20 grams of net carbs per day. What does that look like? For each one of us, it will look slightly different. The end goal is for each day's carb intake to be just 20 grams and for it to be from healthy carbs. How you do it is up to you.

With that in mind, look at this short list of common foods and their corresponding carb count:

- Potato (1 large, baked): 56 grams
- Rice (1 cup, white or brown): 50 grams
- Oatmeal (1 cup, dry): 49 grams
- Pinto beans (1 cup, cooked): 45 grams
- Bagel (whole): 44 grams
- Corn (1 cup, cooked): 41 grams
- Spaghetti (1 cup): 40 grams
- Pizza (1 slice, cheese): 39 grams
- Sweet potato (1 large): 28 grams
- Orange juice (1 cup): 26 grams
- Waffle (1 medium size): 25 grams
- English muffin (whole): 25 grams
- Banana (1 medium): 24 grams
- Apple (1 medium): 21 grams
- Milk (1 cup): 12 grams
- Bread (1 slice, white): 12 grams
- Strawberries (1 cup): 11 grams
- Zucchini (1 medium): 4 grams

- Egg (1 large): 0.6 grams[1]

The saying "an apple a day keeps the doctor away" may have some truth to it, but it will also be almost your total net carbs for the day. A medium apple, speaking of average apples, contains about 20 grams of carbs, with about 3 grams of fiber, which means the net carbs for that medium apple are going to be about 17 grams. Yes, they may be healthy carbs, but they still count against your daily amount.

A baked potato? A cup of cooked pinto beans? A single slice of cheese pizza? A cup of rice? A bagel? Forget it. Each of these is about twice the number of carbs that you need per day for your body to be burning fat in a keto diet.

While you are trying to lose weight or fight sickness or disease, you simply need to choose other low-carb foods. That's all there is to it. I suggest getting your daily carbs from your salad greens, vegetables, limited amounts of low-sugar fruits (such as berries), and nuts. You need those anyway in your keto diet.

Later, when you are at your desired weight and/or have achieved your health goals and you shift over to the Mediterranean-keto lifestyle, you will be able eat more carbs.

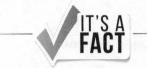

Of the three macronutrients that food contains—fat, protein, and carbohydrates—only carbs are nonessential.

For now, it's understandably more restrictive. But never forget that the end goal is your goal.

With your daily limit of 20 grams of healthy net carbs, divide that into the meals you do eat. You will be surprised how well it can work. For example, let's say your breakfast includes one egg over easy and half a cup of cooked spinach sprinkled with a little feta cheese and drizzled with 2 tablespoons of olive oil. All of that adds up to about 2 grams of net carbs in total.

If for lunch you had chicken-avocado lettuce wraps (consisting of half an avocado, 1 tablespoon of avocado mayo, lemon juice, 6 ounces of chicken breast, several lettuce leaves, a half cup of chopped walnuts, spices, and drizzled with 2 tablespoons of olive oil), that would be around 6 grams of net carbs.

And for dinner if you chose salmon with asparagus (consisting of 6 ounces of salmon fillet, about seven asparagus spears, grated Parmesan cheese, spices, and drizzled with 2 tablespoons of olive oil), you would be at about 4 grams of net carbs.

In short, after three meals like this, you are only at 12 grams of net carbs for the day, and all of these are healthy carbs. (More food choices and recipes are listed in the back of this book.) Thankfully, there is no shortage of delicious menu options when it comes to a keto diet and keeping your daily net carbs to 20 grams or less.

And there are even more options when you do shift over to the Mediterranean-keto lifestyle. There, you will have 50–100 grams of carbs to play with each day, depending on your goals, weight, exercise habits, and so forth.

Remember, we go through the tighter keto diet to get us to the more relaxed Mediterranean-keto lifestyle, where we can live and thrive.

MAKE YOUR CARBS COUNT

As a recap, here are some of the many initial benefits that come from a keto diet:

- appetite control
- weight loss
- increased energy
- more mental clarity
- greater focus

These benefits, and the many others that come from a healthy keto diet, are the direct result of the food choices you make at this point.

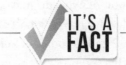

There are many keto calculator options to choose from. This is one that I like and often recommend to my patients: https://calculo.io/keto-calculator.

I tell patients all the time to keep their motivation and goals in mind: "Why are you here?" That is usually a strong enough motivator to help them press through the times when they have to choose less fun, less sweet, or less habitual foods.

As you are carefully counting your carbs, this is the time when adding in what you learned in previous chapters will make things click. All the pieces come together. For example, remember the three vitally important additions to a keto diet:

1. vegetables

2. fiber

3. omega-3

Eating more vegetables and more fiber has been proven to be necessary and beneficial, and this is when you do it. You also watch for opportunities to eat omega-3-rich foods, as well as take omega-3 supplements.

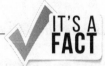

Whole wheat bread is worse for you in causing weight gain than plain sugar because it contains wheat germ agglutinin (WGA) in the bran. WGA is a lectin that behaves similarly to insulin, causing weight gain and eventually insulin resistance.[2]

Since your carb intake is so limited, you are forced to make them count. Do research. Find options. Try new things. For example, low-sugar, low-starch vegetables must obviously top your list, as vegetables (especially salads) are an important part of a healthy keto diet. You will quickly learn which vegetables will help you hit your 20 grams of net carbs per day and which will set you back.

And if you are looking for low-sugar fruits, you will find that black-berries, blueberries, raspberries, and strawberries are healthy, tasty, and lower in sugar than the typical banana, apple, or orange. You may even want to try green bananas, as they have much less sugar than a ripe banana.

How about low-carb sweeteners? There are so many options besides sugar (beet sugar, cane sugar, etc.) or artificial (and often toxic) sweeteners. Those include sweeteners such as erythritol, inulin, monk fruit, stevia, tagatose, and xylitol.[3] There are even low-carb, gluten-free flours that you can use, such as almond flour, coconut flour, flaxseed meal, psyllium husk powder, and walnut and macadamia nut flours.

This is also the time when you read the fine print! There are sugars hidden in virtually everything—sauces, condiments (especially ketchup), nut butters (especially peanut butter), spices, and more—that will ruin your carb counting and your efforts for the day. Just 1 tablespoon of ketchup contains 1 teaspoon of sugar.

This is also the time when you remember to:

- decrease inflammation (less saturated fats especially)

- avoid toxins

- watch alcohol intake carefully

It all comes into play as you are choosing the carbs you eat. After all, carbs determine the overall effectiveness of your keto diet.

The strict carb limit of 20 grams of net carbs is ideal for losing weight and burning off unwanted fat. It's also the key that unlocks the entire keto diet. Without the low-carb intake, there is no keto diet.

Again, perfection is not required. Do your best as you work toward your health goals. In no time, you will begin to notice and count carbs with ease.

And now that you better understand carbs, you are more prepared for healthy living!

Chapter 11

ARE YOU IN KETOSIS?

KETOSIS IS SIMPLE and yet complicated, all rolled into one. To most people on a keto diet, ketosis is simply that sweet spot where they lose weight. But ketosis is much more than that.

WHAT IS KETOSIS?

Ketosis is that healthy and natural state where your body is burning fat for fuel rather than burning sugar for fuel. The standard high-carb American diet burns glucose, or sugar, while a low-carb keto diet burns fats as fuel. When your metabolism shifts from sugar burning to fat burning, that is ketosis.

WHAT MAKES KETOSIS HAPPEN?

Ketosis happens when you reduce your carbs to around 5–15 percent of your daily food intake. Some people may need to go even lower than 5 percent, but usually 5–15 percent is low enough for ketosis to occur.

HOW DOES KETOSIS BENEFIT YOU?

It is the state of ketosis that provides you with the benefits of a keto diet. The many benefits of a keto diet stem from the fact that you got your body into ketosis, where you can enjoy

- weight loss
- increased energy
- mental clarity
- lower blood pressure

89

- clearer skin

- lower inflammation in your body

- controlled food cravings

- lower risk of cancer

- reduced and even eliminated seizures

- reduced or reversed PCOS (polycystic ovary syndrome)

- improved or reversed type 2 diabetes.[1]

HOW LONG DOES IT TAKE TO REACH KETOSIS?

If you are healthy, ketosis will usually occur within two to seven days after you lower your carbs to around 5–15 percent of your daily food intake. If you are insulin resistant, prediabetic, or diabetic, it may take longer (often four to eight weeks) to enter ketosis. Rest assured, you will eventually reach ketosis.

HOW DO YOU FEEL IN KETOSIS?

Pay attention to your body as you eventually shift into ketosis. Try to listen to how your body feels. Here are six common feelings that most people in ketosis have:

1. You should feel satisfied throughout the day because fat and protein burn more slowly than carbs.

2. You should feel like you have a steady supply of energy rather than the ups and downs throughout the day that carbs offer.

3. You should feel more mentally focused because your blood-sugar levels are usually under better control.

4. You should feel in control of your appetite (rather than it controlling you) because the hunger hormone (ghrelin) is no longer telling you, "I'm starving!"

5. You may feel like you can skip a meal because you still feel satisfied several hours after your last meal.

6. You should feel lighter because you are losing weight!

HOW LONG CAN YOU STAY IN KETOSIS?

You can remain in ketosis as long as you like. It's healthy. I recommend that you stay in the fat-burning state of ketosis until you reach your desired weight or have treated any sickness or disease you are fighting. Then shift over to the Mediterranean-keto lifestyle.

WILL KETOSIS BURN YOUR BODY OUT EVENTUALLY?

Our bodies usually have more than 40,000 calories stored away as fat and around 2,000 calories stored in carbohydrate form as glycogen in the liver and muscles (approximately 400 calories in the liver and about 1,600 calories in the muscles), so there is no risk that being in ketosis will burn you out.[2] What's more, the foods you eat will continue to provide your body with more fuel, so ketosis can continue indefinitely.

HOW DO YOU KNOW YOU ARE IN KETOSIS?

As I said, if your daily carbohydrate intake is down around 20 grams, then you will eventually be in ketosis, usually in two to seven days if you are not insulin resistant. If you are insulin resistant, it may take you four to eight weeks before you enter ketosis. If you feel like you are in ketosis and have the positive symptoms that match, then you are probably in ketosis. If you are losing weight, then you really most likely are in ketosis. You can also take a test that will measure the ketones in your system.

HOW DO YOU TEST FOR KETOSIS?

When your body is in ketosis, it burns fat, which is converted in your liver to ketones. These ketones are carbon compounds made in the liver from the breakdown of fat that your body uses for fuel, and they come in three different forms:

- acetone (which you can measure in your breath)

- acetoacetate (which you can measure in your urine)

- beta-hydroxybutyrate (which you can measure in your blood)

The actual number or measurement of ketones in your body will be around 0.5 to 3.0 millimolar (mM) when you are in ketosis and you measure with a blood ketone meter (which is similar to a blood glucose meter). Interestingly, for the first month or two of ketosis, you can usually test all three ketones (with a breathalyzer, urine test strips, and a blood test meter), but after that only the beta-hydroxybutyrate ketone remains accurately measurable. To do so, you will need a blood ketone meter.

IS KETOSIS TESTING REQUIRED?

In a very short amount of time, you will begin to get a feel for being in ketosis. Almost everyone does. But if you want to test for ketones as you are getting used to your keto diet, then do it. I usually recommend the urine test strips, as they are inexpensive, easy to use, and effective for the first month. After that you'll need a blood test meter. The blood test strips for these blood meters are not as cheap as the urine test strips, but they are the most accurate way to measure ketones.

Most people, however, don't like to track their ketones. That's fine. But if that's you, pay extra careful attention to your body, how you feel, what you eat, and so on. You are tuning your internal ear to know when you are in ketosis. That's good, as this ability will benefit you for the rest of your life.

HOW LONG SHOULD YOU TRACK KETOSIS?

For patients with cancer, obesity, sickness, or disease, I do recommend that they test for ketones for the first three to six months on a keto diet. That helps, as shifting into ketosis is often a little more difficult with health-related issues. For healthy people during the first four to six weeks of a keto diet, it is handy to be able to test (especially urine test strips) for ketones, but if they get a feel for it and don't want to test, that's fine. It's entirely up to you.

WHAT BUMPS YOU OUT OF KETOSIS?

As long as your carb intake is down around 5 percent or about 20 grams per day, you should remain in ketosis. This is similar to what might cause your weight loss to plateau (from chapter 7). That is because there are only a limited number of reasons your body will not be in ketosis, and they all have to do with the macronutrient break-down for your daily food intake on your keto diet:

- 75 percent fats
- 20 percent proteins
- 5 percent carbs

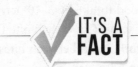

Signs of insulin resistance:

- Hemoglobin A1C of 5.7 or greater
- Fasting triglyceride level over 150 milligrams per deciliter
- HDL cholesterol level under 40 milligrams per deciliter in men, 50 milligrams per deciliter in women
- Waistline over 40 inches in men, 35 inches in women
- Fasting glucose over 100 milligrams per deciliter

Here are five of the most common causes for people bumping themselves out of ketosis:

1. Not consuming enough fat (the goal is 75 percent)—
   This is often a lack of olive oil, but make sure you are
   getting the right amount of fats per meal per day. For a
   woman on 1,600 calories a day, that is 10 tablespoons
   of fat a day, or 3.33 tablespoons per meal. For men, it's
   about 15 tablespoons a day, or 5 tablespoons per meal.

2. Eating too much protein (the goal is 20 percent)—
   Remember, if you eat too much protein, the extra protein converts to sugar.

3. Eating too many carbs (the goal is 5 percent)—This is
   only 20 grams a day or equivalent to 1.5 slices of bread.
   It's not much, so monitor your carb intake carefully for
   a few days. Also, watch for those carbs that can sneak
   in with nut butters, artificial sweeteners, and sauces.

4. Eating too much (practice eating until satisfied)—Dial
   back your total food intake by 5–10 percent. That will
   adjust all your macros. Chew each bite twenty to thirty
   times. Put your fork down between bites, and enjoy
   good conversation with family.

5. Unexpected stressors (be patient, ketosis will kick in)—
   This is often out of your control, but rest assured that
   ketosis will happen. Keep moving forward.

For most people, it's usually too many carbs or not enough fats. These are admittedly the two biggest changes from the standard American diet, so it is understandable that it takes some getting used to. Keep going, keep your macros in line, and your body will follow your lead.

HOW IS KETOSIS A LIFESTYLE?

Fat-burning is a lifestyle that everyone wants. But not many people are willing to stay on a strict keto diet for years and years, even if it is a constant fat-burning machine. This is the time, whether it has been three months or three years, when many people revert back to their old high-carb diet.

As we have discussed, that can bring about some very bad results, especially if they have been eating too many saturated fats on their keto diet and then mix that with a high-carb diet.

The answer, and the goal all along, is to shift over from the keto diet to the Mediterranean-keto lifestyle or to rotate between the healthy keto diet and the Mediterranean-keto lifestyle. It's a natural transition.

When you have used a healthy keto diet to get your body where you want it to be, whether it's losing weight or fighting some sickness or disease, it's time to move over to the Mediterranean-keto lifestyle.

In the Mediterranean-keto lifestyle, the macronutrients look more like this:

- 50–55 percent fats
- 20–25 percent proteins
- 20–25 percent carbs

You can tweak them yourself as you go to maintain your own health goals, but here is the beauty of it: your body usually continues to burn fat rather than sugar. Your body adjusted to ketosis (as our bodies naturally do) and became efficient at it.

With the Mediterranean-keto lifestyle of low carbs, high healthy fats, and moderate proteins (like a keto diet, just relaxed a bit), your body will cycle in and out of ketosis. To me it's like a flying fish; it lives in the ocean yet it can glide over the waves for long distances, then land back in the water, and then zoom out again.

Your body will continue to burn fat as its main fuel source. Some days more so, some days less, but you continue to control the fat-burning engine by what you eat. That is how ketosis can be a lifestyle.

Ketosis is where it's at. That's where the action is. On a pretty strict keto diet, your body will basically remain in the state of ketosis, morning, noon, and night.

When you shift over to the Mediterranean-keto lifestyle, you will drift in and out of ketosis. You will still get the health benefits and some of the weight loss benefits of a keto diet, but things will be more relaxed in your food regimen. (We will talk more about the specifics in the coming chapters.) Ketosis is the healthiest place that your body can be. As a diet and then as a lifestyle, it makes perfect sense.

Chapter 12

HOW TO BEAT THE KETO FLU

THE KETO FLU is not a flu. Rather, it's a combination of non-life-threatening symptoms that feel like a flu. That's all. And for the most part, it's your body's reaction to shifting from a high-carb diet to a low-carb diet.

You could call it withdrawal if you want, but these symptoms are common to almost everyone starting on a keto diet. They often occur at the beginning right as you are trying to shift from sugar-burning to fat-burning.

During the shift, as you are purposefully decreasing the sugars, carbs, and starches and increasing the fat intake, there is often a gap where there is less-than-normal energy on hand to burn. It's like the doldrums, where there is no wind and the sailing ships are stuck. You have lowered your carbs to only 20 grams but have not shifted into ketosis so that you are burning fats effectively. You simply don't have enough carbs to maintain your energy needs.

But you can rest assured that these symptoms will eventually pass away, sometimes within minutes, hours, or days. Either way, they usually don't last long once you learn the simple solutions for keto flu, which I will discuss shortly.

THE KETO FLU

Here is a collection of keto flu symptoms, many of which came from my patients over the years:

- fatigue
- headache
- brain fog (example: locking your keys in the car)

- frequent urination

- trouble sleeping

- diarrhea

- weakness

- irritability

- muscle cramps

- lethargy

- dehydration

- nausea

- hunger

- light-headedness

- forgetfulness

- constipation

- bad breath

- lack of focus

- gas[1]

Naturally, nobody wants these symptoms. After all, it usually feels like you have come down with the flu without the fever! The answer is to cross over into ketosis as quickly as you can.

You may be wondering, Is what bumps you out of ketosis (from chapter 11) also what keeps you from reaching ketosis? Yes, for the most part, that is usually the case. So if you have keto flu symptoms, examine your food intake. Determine if you are getting enough fats (75 percent of your daily intake), eating too much protein (over 20 percent), or eating too many carbs (over 5 percent or more than 20 grams of carbs per day).

Most often if you can get the three macronutrient proportions correct, it will usually be enough to get you out of the keto flu doldrums and into ketosis. Some, however, will need salt, more water, electrolytes, or exogenous ketones to overcome the keto flu.

EXTRA HELP TO GET ACROSS

Everyone is different. For those who are healthy and take just a few days to shift into ketosis, they may not experience keto flu at all. Or the symptoms may be mild. For those who are obese, prediabetic, type 2 diabetic, insulin resistant, fighting cancer, or suffering from some other sickness, it can take several weeks (four to eight) to shift into ketosis. And the symptoms may be more pronounced and last for days or weeks.

For some of us, our bodies have been burning sugar as fuel for forty or fifty years, even seventy or eighty years! It's simply going to take a little time for the shift to happen. There are a lot of changes, reverses, and revisions involved in the process. It's not an instant process.

With that said, it does not mean you have to soldier on and press through, regardless of the pain. Yes, to a certain degree we all have to press through, but if there is an answer that eases the pain or speeds up the shift to ketosis, then let's do it!

Here are several things you can do to help yourself past any keto flu symptoms and into ketosis more quickly.

Add more salt.

We all have about 4 pounds of water that is retained in our bodies due to salt and insulin. It is there because of the high amounts of insulin our bodies use to balance the high-carb food intake. In other words, a high-carb diet causes higher insulin levels, which causes us to retain water.

But when you lower your carbs on a keto diet, this water is released, which is why you have about a four-pound weight loss the first week on a keto diet. Along with the water goes the sodium that has been retained due to the higher insulin levels. In other words, the lower insulin levels have a direct effect on the body initially.

Many of the keto flu symptoms are a direct result of low sodium.

Thankfully, the answer is simple enough: add more sodium to your diet.

You can boost your sodium by

- adding ½ to 1 teaspoon sea salt or Himalayan pink salt to a glass of water

- adding 1 bouillon cube to a cup of warm water

- eating a bowl of healthy, low-carb soup

- eating salty pickled vegetables

- salting your food more than usual.

You need about 2–5 grams of salt per day (1 teaspoon is 5 grams of salt), and more if you are active (i.e., sweating a lot outside). I like to use the pink Himalayan salt, but sea salt and kosher salt are great as well. Start low (at ½ teaspoon of salt) and go slow if you have hypertension, and monitor your blood pressure.

Feel free to salt pretty much all your foods, even your drinks. If you have keto flu symptoms, and have already made sure you are on target with your macronutrient amounts (75 percent fat, 20 percent protein, 5 percent carb), then low sodium is the most likely culprit.

Drink more water.

The second most likely culprit behind keto flu symptoms is dehydration. Interestingly, lack of water and low sodium cause almost the exact same keto flu symptoms, but it makes sense when you see how they are connected.

On a keto diet, now that insulin levels are lower, water is not retained as it once was. Because sodium is stored in the intracellular and extracellular fluids within your body, when your fluid levels go down, your sodium levels also go down.

You will need to drink more water, but don't overdo it. Why not? Because more water will dilute the sodium in your system (increasing the keto flu symptoms), and more water intake will cause you to go to the bathroom more frequently (and out goes the sodium), which may make things even worse. When you are thirsty, drink. That's the most practical middle ground when it comes to your fluid levels to prevent dehydration but also add back some salt.

Add electrolytes.

Sodium is not the only electrolyte (a mineral that carries an electric charge) that can go low while your body is recalibrating itself. In addition to sodium, people may become deficient in magnesium, calcium, chloride, phosphorus, and potassium. In fact, 50–90 percent of people are deficient in magnesium.[2]

Water does not have these electrolytes, but you can get them from the foods you eat. Here is a list of electrolytes and foods that contain them:

- potassium (avocados, nuts, dark leafy greens, salmon, and mushrooms)

- magnesium (nuts, dark chocolate, artichokes, spinach)

- calcium (leafy greens, broccoli, seafood, almonds)

- phosphorus (meats, nuts, seeds, dark chocolate)

- chloride (most veggies, olives, salt, seaweed)[3]

An electrolyte drink is also a great way to quickly raise your electrolyte levels.

Take psyllium husk powder.

During the shift from burning sugar for fuel to burning fat for fuel, there are several areas in your body where there is a lot of action taking place. The gut is one of those places.

One of the best calming agents for the gut is fiber in the form of psyllium husk powder. Your body needs at least 2 tablespoons of this fiber per day, but you need to work up to that amount. I suggest starting at 1 teaspoon once in the morning after breakfast and once after dinner before bed, slowly working up to 1 tablespoon or more twice a day.

Just because people are starting a keto diet does not erase these facts:

- Only 5 percent of Americans consume enough fiber.[4]

- Constipation usually worsens with age, and more than forty million adults in the United States (about 16 percent of the population) suffer from chronic constipation.[5]

- Millions of people in the United States have acid reflux and take antacids, which usually increase constipation.[6]

What's more, several of the typical keto flu symptoms, such as diarrhea, constipation, dehydration, and gas, are helped by the psyllium husk powder. The psyllium husk powder also helps you achieve your health goals because it makes you feel satisfied longer (thus controlling appetite), slows digestion, normalizes bowel movements, increases insulin sensitivity, gives you energy, and improves your metabolism.

THE SUGAR CYCLE

We all know the sugar cycle. We have all experienced it:

1. Eat sugar (carbs, sugar, etc.)
2. Dopamine released (the happy hormone)
3. Insulin secreted to lower blood-sugar levels
4. Insulin rises, blood-sugar level lowers, body crashes
5. Hungry, want more sugar
6. Repeat[7]

The problem is that coming off carbs and sugar is like coming off a drug. Sugar addicts not only have similar behavior to substance abusers but they also have "similar neurochemical and brain activation patterns."[8] Our favorite foods aren't called comfort foods for nothing. We are often addicted to them. We want them. We need them! And if we don't get them, we experience withdrawals, which match the keto flu symptoms. But press on. You will eventually come out on the other side. And you will have broken the sugar cycle in your body and in your brain.

Add MCT oil/powder.

One supplement that needs to be part of your keto diet and eventual Mediterranean-keto lifestyle is MCT oil. MCT stands for medium-chain triglyceride, and it comes in powder, liquid, or capsule form. I recommend the powder form of MCT oil because it is perfect for stirring into coffee or tea. (It also comes in several flavors; see the supplements section for more information.)

MCT oil is very effective at pushing you into ketosis. It's like a strong gust of wind that helps blow you out of the keto flu doldrums. With your coffee or tea, start with 1–2 teaspoons. Start low with MCT oil as it can cause loose stools. Slowly increase the amount, but I'd not suggest more than 1 tablespoon of MCT oil at a time. MCT oil tends to cause loose stools in many, but MCT oil powder is less likely to cause loose stools.

Moderate MCT oil consumption is a healthy addition to your daily routine. And as you begin a keto diet, it is especially beneficial because it helps propel you forward into ketosis. And once that occurs, MCT is more good fuel to your fat-burning fire.

Take exogenous ketones.

Though it sounds exotic, exogenous ketones are simply supplements of the ketone beta-hydroxybutyrate, which your body makes when you are on a low-carb keto diet. They are ketone salts, including sodium beta-hydroxybutyrate, magnesium beta-hydroxybutyrate, potassium beta-hydroxybutyrate, and calcium beta-hydroxybutyrate. These really tend to pull most people out of keto flu, usually within thirty minutes to an hour.

These ketones, whether from your own body or as a supplement, efficiently and effectively raise your blood ketone levels so you start burning fat for fuel right away, and that means you are in ketosis.[9]

They also help control hunger, increase your energy levels, boost your mental capacity, and relieve keto flu symptoms.

As a supplement, these exogenous ketones are like MCT oil, only stronger. They can help you be in ketosis usually within the hour. I usually recommend exogenous ketones to people who are insulin resistant, are prediabetic, have type 2 diabetes, or are obese, as their bodies typically need an extra boost to get over to ketosis. But for anyone wanting to get into ketosis more quickly, exogenous ketones are ideal. (See appendix A, "Recommended Supplements," for more information.) They also help rescue patients from keto flu because they contain the key ketone salts (sodium, potassium, magnesium, and calcium beta-hydroxybutyrate). Personally, I take exogenous ketones before a workout. They give me more energy. You can do the same if you want, but for now use these ketones to help you get into ketosis and out of the keto flu.

DON'T CUT CORNERS

While people are shifting from sugar-burning to fat-burning, they are tempted to do whatever it takes to get their bodies out of the doldrums and into ketosis. They are tempted to cut corners, so to speak, in an effort to either handle the unpleasant keto flu symptoms or to try to push themselves into fat-burning more quickly.

I get it, but the fastest and surest way to reach ketosis and past any keto flu symptoms is by applying the previous help options. They work and have worked for thousands of people. With that said, following are several corners that you do not want to cut.

- **Don't eat sugar.** Sugar withdrawals are normal, but consuming sweets, such as a donut or soda, will pull you backward rather than forward. Eat no-sugar dark chocolate. It will boost your dopamine (the happy hormone) levels without slowing you down.

- **Don't undereat.** This is not the time to starve yourself. Continue to eat and drink in line with your body's macronutrient proportions.

- **Don't drink excess water.** This may help with headaches, but too much water at this time will deplete your salt levels (see Help #1). Just drink when you are thirsty.

- **Don't do a detox program.** The shift to a low-carb diet is in itself a detox program as your body releases toxins that have been stored in fat. Doing a detox will not help alleviate the keto flu symptoms; it may only make matters worse. Just keep going, and apply all the help options.

- **Don't exercise excessively.** Light exercise (such as walking) is always good, but more exercise or increasing your exercise intensity will not help you with your keto flu symptoms or push you through to ketosis. Exercise at this time may in fact make you feel even worse. Feel free to keep doing a light exercise routine, but don't add extra exercise.

WILL THE KETO FLU RETURN?

Experiencing keto flu symptoms once is bad enough, but will they ever come back? That's a good question, and the answer is maybe. Let me explain.

Once you reach ketosis and that has become your new normal, there are usually only two main reasons that you might feel those same keto flu symptoms again. The first reason is what you would expect: eating too many carbs. If you eat more carbs than your own level of fat-burning can handle, you will be bumped out of ketosis, and keto flu symptoms may return. Brain fog, lethargy, and feeling unfocused are most common.

You already know the solution to the problem: decrease your carb intake.

If you do eat more carbohydrates than your macronutrient levels allow (it's best not to), try to do it for dinner. Then you will usually sleep well. If you do it at lunch, you may need to take a nap in the middle of the day! Either way, the next day is a new day. Jump back into your planned keto diet routine.

The second reason that you may experience keto flu symptoms again is less expected: too much exercise. Our bodies burn glucose when running or during intense exercise. The problem is that your body is purposefully very low in glucose, and your glycogen stores (stored in your muscles and liver) are probably depleted because you are burning fat for fuel. If there is not enough glucose on hand for intense exercise, your body will not like it.[10]

I experienced this firsthand. After intense workouts, I would usually crash and need a thirty-minute nap. I thought something was wrong with me, but I had forgotten that short bursts of exercise (as is common in intense workouts, running, bicycling, high cardio training, or physical outdoor work) burn glucose. It's best not to do intense exercise until you reach your goal weight, then increase your carbs before your workouts.

The answer is to eat more carbs on the days that you do more intense exercise. For athletes, they simply need to eat more carbs on the days that they train.

Eating small to moderate amounts of fruit, sweet potatoes, beans, rice, and other healthy carbs is good before you do high-intensity exercise. Learn to find the balance, and build that into your routine so you don't have a relapse of the keto flu.

Thankfully, the keto flu passes. It is not a permanent condition in the slightest. In time, it will be a distant memory.

Chapter 13

SEVEN STEPS TO STARTING YOUR KETO DIET

I T'S TIME TO set up your healthy keto diet so that you can dive in and begin the process. There is much to remember, so this chapter is purposefully straightforward and step-by-step. In the very forefront are the macronutrient levels for your healthy keto diet:

- 75 percent fats

- 20 percent proteins

- 5 percent carbs

Everything builds on that. When you feel you are ready and shift over to the Mediterranean-keto lifestyle, everything will build on those new macronutrient numbers.

STEPS FOR STARTING YOUR KETO DIET

Basically, you are going from where you are to where you want to be. That is point A to point B. And along the way your health goals are your constant source of motivation.

Step-by-step this is where your keto diet begins:

Step 1: Define your starting point.
These are the action steps to take:

- Weigh yourself on a scale.

- Take photos (optional).

- Take body measurements (optional).

Record this information in a journal, on your phone, or somewhere that works for you. Defining your starting point may not feel important at the moment, but it will prove to be a valuable source of information as you move forward. It may also be a source of encouragement as you lose weight.

Step 2: Do the math.

These are the action steps to take:

1. Decrease total daily food intake by about 20 percent.

2. Apply your macronutrient levels:

   * 75 percent fats

   * 20 percent proteins

   * 5 percent carbs

3. Calculate your calories per macro.

4. Convert calories to grams per macro.

For women

The average adult woman in the United States consumes around 1,600–2,400 calories in food per day. To lose weight, you want to decrease that to 1,600 calories per day while maintaining your healthy keto diet macros. (A 20 percent decrease in daily food intake is usually sufficient to cause weight loss, but 1,600 calories per day is a great starting point.)

Using the macro levels and 1,600 calories, that means

- 1,200 calories from fats

- 320 calories from proteins

- 80 calories from carbs.

For men

The average adult male in the United States consumes around twenty-four hundred to 3,800 calories in food per day. To lose weight, you should decrease your food intake to 2,000–2,400 calories per day while maintaining your healthy keto diet macros. (A 20 percent decrease in daily food intake is usually sufficient to cause weight loss, but 2,000–2,400 calories per day is a great starting point.)

Using the macro levels and 2,400 calories, that means

- 1,800 calories from fats

- 480 calories from proteins

- 120 calories from carbs.

According to the USDA, the calories-to-grams ratio for fats is 9 calories per 1 gram of fat, 4 calories per 1 gram of protein, and 4 calories per 1 gram of carbs. Doing the math for women at 1,600 calories per day, that is

- 133 grams fats

- 80 grams proteins

- 20 grams carbs.

For men at 2,400 calories per day, that is

- 200 grams fats

- 120 grams proteins

- 30 grams carbs. (I still usually start men on 20 grams carbs.)

Most people have no idea what their daily caloric intake is. If you want to track your calories for a day or two to give yourself a baseline, that is fine. Or you can simply choose a starting point (i.e., 1,600 calories for women, 2,000–2,400 calories for men) and begin. For most people, that is sufficient.

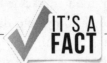

- 1 gram of fat = 9 calories
- 1 gram of carbs = 4 calories
- 1 gram of protein = 4 calories

For obese or bigger people, I often recommend that they decrease by 20 percent for two to four weeks, then decrease by another 20 percent, and so on, until they eventually reach the sixteen hundred (for women) or two thousand to twenty-four hundred (for men) threshold. This creates more of a gradual weight loss plan.

You decide on your caloric intake per day. Whatever that starting point number is for you, begin there.

Step 3: Approximate your foods.
These are the action steps to take:

- Approximate grams per macronutrient per meal.

- Practice calculating macro amounts using real foods.

For women at 1,600 calories eating three meals per day, that means approximately

- 44 grams fats per meal (around 3.33 tablespoons fats per meal)

- 27 grams proteins per meal (around 4 ounces proteins per meal)

- 7 grams carbs per meal.

For men at 2,400 calories eating three meals per day, that means approximately

- 67 grams fats per meal (around 5 tablespoons fats per meal)

- 40 grams proteins per meal (around 6 ounces proteins per meal)

- 10 grams carbs per meal (or 7 grams per meal if you choose 20 grams carbs per day).

If you are starting at a different calories-per-day point than these, that's fine. Just make sure you know what your daily goal is and divide that by your intended number of meals per day. For most people, I would recommend three meals per day to begin and later, once you reach nutritional ketosis, you can practice intermittent fasting and eat just two meals a day in an eight-hour window of time.

Once you have your approximate grams per macro per meal figured out, it's time to start practicing. For example, a large egg has these approximate macronutrient numbers: 5 grams of fat, 6 grams of protein, and 0.6 grams of carbs.

So, for example, let's say for breakfast you had

- 2 eggs (10 grams fat, 12 grams protein, 1 gram carbs)

- 2 thin slices of turkey bacon (4.5 grams fat, 4.7 grams protein, 0.5 grams carbs)

- ½ medium tomato (0.1 grams fat, 0.5 grams protein, 2.4 grams carbs)

- 1 medium avocado (24 grams fat, 3 grams protein, 3 grams carbs)

- Totals: 38.6 grams fat, 20.2 grams protein, 6.9 grams carbs.

From this example breakfast, a woman eating 1,600 calories in a day would be almost on target for fats per meal, a little shy on proteins per meal, and on target for carbs per meal. She would need to add a little more protein, maybe as a snack (e.g., nuts) later in the morning.

For a man eating 2,400 calories in a day, this breakfast would get him only partway there. He would especially need more fats and proteins, but the carbs are still about right.

Begin to practice figuring out the macros (fats, proteins, and carbs) with healthy foods and using that information per meal.

Thankfully all this math and these calculations per food and recipes have already been figured out. It's good to be able to find out (online especially) what the macronutrients are per food item, but you don't have to build your entire recipe list on your own (unless you want to).

There are many keto recipes out there. Included in part 3 of this book are several recipes for starting a Mediterranean-keto lifestlye, including several strictly keto meal ideas that will help you as you begin your healthy keto weight loss journey.

Step 4: Choose your meals.

These are the action steps to take:

- Choose the meals you want to eat.

- Make sure the macronutrients are met per meal.

With so many keto recipes available, whether online or in the back of this book, you simply need to choose the meals you want to eat that match what you need for your macronutrient amounts per meal. Start with basic and easy meals, with lots of salads. The more you plan ahead and prepare, the less spontaneous you will need to be—and it's very hard to be spontaneous and hit your macronutrient goals when you are doing something new.

Later on, after you get a feel for your ketosis and food counts, you can be more creative and last-minute in your meals. But for now it's better (and easier on you) to plan ahead. I suggest planning ahead for a full week. That way you can shop in advance and won't have to think so much about it.

Don't worry, you will get a hang of this as you go!

Step 5: Restock your fridge and pantry.

These are the action steps to take:

- Clean out what you don't want.

- Restock with what you do want.

This is often a light-bulb moment, one of those aha moments when people realize what they've been eating. When you look at the foods in your pantry, you may do the same. For example,

- one regular bagel: 1 gram fat, 9 grams protein, 55 grams carbs

- one cup 2 percent milk: 4.8 grams fat, 8 grams protein, 12 grams carbs

- one large banana: 0.5 grams fat, 1.5 grams protein, 31 grams carbs

- one cup cooked oatmeal: 3.6 grams fat, 5.9 grams protein, 28 grams carbs.

Quite often the moment you count the carbs in something, you know immediately whether it's an option.

No matter how healthy something might be, while you are on a healthy keto diet, you simply need to stick to your fat, protein, and carb macronutrient numbers. That's going to require you to clean certain things out of your fridge and pantry and replace them with healthy low-carb, medium-protein, and high-fat options.

You can spend the time doing the calculations per item in your fridge and pantry, but in the end you will find pretty much that everything that is in a box, bag, or can has too many carbs in it or the fats are unhealthy. Out go the breads, cereals, baked goods, oats, pasta (of any sort), rice, potatoes, flour (regular and wheat), sugar (liquid, granulated, or powder), creamers, cookies, ice cream, syrups, sodas, juices, granola bars, oils (vegetable, canola, soybean), margarine, alcohol, and so on. Even dried fruits like cranberries, raisins, and dates or raw fruits like bananas, grapes, oranges, and mangoes need to go.

When in doubt, look up the food item and see what the macronutrient numbers are to see if it fits with your healthy keto diet plans. If you have beans, peas, or lentils in bags, you can put those on a back shelf for later. When you shift over to the Mediterranean-keto lifestyle, you will want these items again.

In place of these items, you will want to restock your fridge and pantry with foods that fit your healthy keto diet. These same items will also fit the Mediterranean-keto lifestyle, so doing this now will help you in the future. They will also work with the keto recipes in this book and others you find.

Following is a good base of what should be in your fridge and pantry. (See appendix D for a complete list.)

- oils—extra-virgin, cold-pressed olive and avocado especially (in dark glass containers); MCT oil (powder or liquid); coconut, almond, walnut, and macadamia oils (preferably cold-pressed)

- vegetables—arugula, cabbage, cucumbers, broccoli, celery, spinach, kale, chard, romaine, artichokes, green beans, Brussels sprouts, olives, radish, cauliflower, greens (collard, mustard, dandelion), asparagus, garlic, mushrooms, onions, yellow squash, zucchini, spaghetti squash, peppers, eggplant, and tomatoes

- low-sugar fruits—strawberries, raspberries, blackberries, blueberries, limes, lemons, plums, clementines, kiwi, cantaloupe, watermelon

- fresh/dried herbs—ginger, oregano, basil, cilantro, parsley, thyme, rosemary, sage, mint, bay leaves, cumin, curry powder, paprika, black pepper, cayenne pepper, red pepper flakes, cinnamon, cardamom, etc.

- nuts/seeds—almonds, walnuts, Brazil nuts, peanuts, pecans, macadamias, cashews, hazelnuts, pine nuts, pistachios, chia, flax, hemp, pumpkin, sesame, etc.

- pickled/fermented foods—unsweetened kefir or yogurt (especially coconut, goat, and sheep), dill pickles, kimchi, sauerkraut, miso, apple cider vinegar, banana peppers, capers, olives, pickled jalapeños, etc.

- condiments—mustard, avocado mayo, pesto, low- or no-sugar hot sauces, sugar-free ketchup, low-carb Italian dressing, red wine vinegar, balsamic vinegar

- meats—pasture-raised poultry and eggs; wild or sustainably harvested fish, shrimp, oysters, etc.; grass-fed beef, bison, pork, sheep, goat, etc.; wild deer, rabbit, elk, turkey bacon, smoked wild salmon, etc. (bacon and sausage one or two times a week)

- dairy (to be limited to less than 10 percent of your total daily fat intake)—feta, grass-fed ghee, grass-fed butter, sour cream, heavy whipping cream, cheese, cream cheese, unsweetened yogurt, almond milk, coconut milk

- broths—chicken, beef, bone

- natural sweeteners—stevia, monk fruit, erythritol, inulin, tagatose, and xylitol

- coffee, tea, and water (filtered) or sparkling water

- fiber (psyllium husk powder)

- dark chocolate (70 percent or higher cacao)

- healthy carbs to be added in the Mediterranean-keto lifestyle—beans (black, green, snap, pinto, red, kidney, garbanzo, lima, navy, white, lupini), lentils, peas (green and black-eyed), sweet potatoes, yams, cassava, taro root, gluten-free bread or gluten-free pasta, basmati white rice, millet bread, low-sugar fruits, and other healthy carbs

- supplements (See appendix A, "Recommended Supplements.")

It will take a little while for this to become a habit, so be patient with yourself. I have found that the more expensive items (i.e., wild fish or grass-fed beef) are foods that we don't eat every day. Oils and vegetables are relatively inexpensive, and these we use daily for fats and healthy carbs.

Step 6: Set up an exercise routine.
These are the action steps to take:

- Decide how much exercise you want to do.

- Make that exercise a habit.

Walking fifteen to twenty minutes per day is a good starting point for everyone on a keto diet. For many, that will be enough for the first few months. It will help with the weight loss and getting the metabolism in line.

For others, that is not enough. They want to do more, such as thirty to forty-five minutes per day. If that is you, that's fine; just remember that intense exercise may be more than your low-carb keto diet can handle, so increasing your carbs or taking exogenous ketones or MCT oil powder may be necessary (as discussed in the last chapter) on those high-intensity exercise days.

Starting low and going slow is recommended, but whatever you wish to do, make sure you build it into your daily and weekly schedule. Quite simply, make it a habit.

Step 7: Measure your progress.
These are the action steps to take: .

- Decide that you will track your macronutrients.

- Track your food intake for at least four weeks.

There is an old saying, "If you can measure it, you can manage it." With your keto diet, that is especially good advice when you are first getting started. It takes twenty-one days to create a habit, so track your food intake for at least your first full month. That means you count the macronutrients of every meal, snack, or beverage.

Some people prefer to continue tracking for six to twelve months, and that can prove to be helpful (especially if weight loss plateaus), but most people don't want to spend the time and effort to track the macronutrients of their food. But for the first month, you really should track carefully. If you can begin to train your mind to think, "Tracking is my friend," it will help you.

What if it takes you longer to reach ketosis? Then you simply need to keep on tracking your macronutrients until at least a week after you reach that point. (Measuring your ketone levels is also helpful at this time.) The whole point of tracking the macronutrients is knowing where you are on your keto journey. After all, the primary reasons for weight loss plateaus and falling out of ketosis: too many carbs, too many proteins, and not enough healthy fats. And how will you know that if you aren't tracking?

After achieving ketosis, a lot of people will continue forward with a "close enough" mindset, and that can work. They are more likely to be in and out of ketosis, and their weight loss is usually more gradual, but it works for them and they get the results they want, more or less. As you would expect, being a little more than "close enough" will get you much better results.

Based on the results of hundreds of patients who have started a keto diet, I have found this common thread: those who track more carefully are almost always going to get better results. They usually reach ketosis more quickly, lose more weight, have shorter weight loss plateaus, and are generally healthier.

How you track is really up to you. Some do it manually, and some prefer apps that help keep them accountable. There are many keto apps and keto calculators to choose from. I often recommend this one as a good starting point: https://calculo.io/keto-calculator.

SUMMARY OF KETO DIET STEPS

These are the seven steps to starting your keto diet:

Step 1: Define your starting point.

Step 2: Do the math.

Step 3: Approximate your foods.

Step 4: Choose your meals.

Step 5: Restock your fridge and pantry.

Step 6: Set up an exercise routine.

Step 7: Measure your progress.

This is the launching point where you jump into your keto diet journey. You are armed with more than enough knowledge. You have a motivating reason for jumping in. You have all that it takes. It's going to be great! Having a keto partner or support group will help many stay on course and achieve their weight loss goals.

––––––––

Congratulations! As you begin, know that you are starting the best, most effective, and healthiest keto diet in existence. The proven results speak for themselves. Here's to your health and your health goals!

And after you achieve your desired weight and other health goals, you are welcome to shift over to the Mediterranean-keto lifestyle. I'll see you there!

Chapter 14

GET THE MOST FROM YOUR KETO DIET

I F SOMEONE HAS a strong family history of Alzheimer's, type 2 diabetes, dementia, heart disease, insulin resistance, or obesity, they are signing up for the exact same thing if they continue with the standard American diet. In fact, if these same people develop prediabetes, type 2 diabetes, or insulin resistance, then they are twice as likely to develop dementia.

Why are you here? Do you have health goals that motivate you to take action, to get on a keto diet, and then to shift over to the Mediterranean-keto lifestyle? You know why you are here, and my sincere hope is that you achieve every one of your health goals. A healthy keto diet is one of the best health moves you can make, and I commend you for it.

On your healthy keto diet so far:

- Are you starting to lose weight?
- Do you have more energy?
- Do you feel satisfied/less hungry throughout the day?
- Has your appetite come under your control?
- Do you need fewer afternoon naps?
- Has your brain fog lifted?
- Do you have greater mental clarity?

If you answered yes to some or all of these questions, then you are doing something right! These are a few of the common results from a healthy keto diet.

Many of the other benefits (decreased inflammation; insulin levels lowered; lower bad cholesterol; raised good cholesterol; blood sugar controlled; lowered risks for dementia, Alzheimer's, type 2 diabetes, and obesity; fighting cancer; and many more) are internal, and you won't know about them until later or until you do testing.

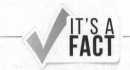

Insulin resistance is a root cause of heart disease, obesity, diabetes, cancer, and dementia, and 88 percent of Americans either have it or significant risk factors for it.[1] And it's 100 percent reversible!

But you can rest assured. Your body benefits on the inside and the outside from a healthy keto diet.

Not every keto diet is healthy. Remember to incorporate the three additions and three subtractions that set a healthy keto diet apart from the rest. These are vital elements of your good health:

1. more vegetables

2. more fiber

3. more omega-3

4. less inflammation (from saturated fats)

5. less toxins

6. less red wine or alcohol (especially if you have the APOE4 gene)

If your weight loss has plateaued, answer these questions:

- Have you eaten too many carbs?

- Are you eating too much protein?

- Are you drinking enough water?
- Have you eaten too many nuts?
- Have you started exercising?
- Have you eaten too much dairy?
- Are you eating enough fat?
- Have you eaten too much food?
- Are you using artificial sweeteners?
- Are you eating hidden sugars?
- Do you need to exercise more?
- Have you tried intermittent fasting?
- Are you experiencing too much stress?
- Are your hormones fluctuating?
- Are you getting enough sleep?
- Is your thyroid sluggish?
- Are you consuming too much sodium?
- Are you exercising too much?

How long have you been on your keto diet? One week? Two weeks? Are you already in ketosis, or is your body taking its good old time getting there? Or maybe you are experiencing keto flu symptoms, such as

- fatigue
- headache
- brain fog
- frequent urination
- trouble sleeping
- diarrhea

- weakness

- irritability

- muscle cramps

- lethargy

- dehydration

- nausea

- hunger

- light-headed

- forgetfulness

- constipation

- bad breath

- unfocused

- gas.

If so, then you may need to

- increase your salt intake

- drink more water

- add electrolytes

- take psyllium husk powder

- add MCT oil/powder

- take exogenous ketones.

If you find your body drifts in and out of ketosis, it may be because you are

- not consuming enough fat (The goal is 75 percent.)

- eating too much protein (The goal is 20 percent.)

- eating too many carbs (The goal is 5 percent or 20 grams a day.)

- eating too much (Practice eating until satisfied.)

- facing unexpected stressors. (Be patient; ketosis will kick in.)

Pay careful attention to the macronutrients in your foods, meals, meal planning, and recipes. For your first month especially, track and measure everything carefully. If it takes you longer to reach ketosis, continue tracking the macronutrients in your food until you do eventually reach ketosis.

KEEP AT IT

If you want to gain the many benefits of a keto diet or have pressing health needs or goals, then you simply must press forward. Keep at it.

If you are thinking of quitting, or have quit already, it's OK. Nobody controls your life. You get to choose your own destiny. My hope, as a medical doctor, is always that you will do all you can to be healthy and live a long life.

Wherever you are on your keto diet, I encourage you to keep your motivating reason for being here right in front of your face at all times. And if you can bring in some of your family, do it. Everything is more fun (and easier to do) when you are part of a team.

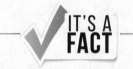

IT'S A
FACT

Olive oil: 1 tablespoon (0.5 ounces) of olive oil (14 grams) contains the following nutritional information, according to the USDA:

- Calories: 119
- Total fat: 13.5 grams

- » Saturated fat: 1.9 grams
- » Polyunsaturated fat: 1.4 grams
- » Monounsaturated fat: 9.9 grams
- » Trans fat: O grams
- Total carbohydrates: O grams
  - » Dietary fiber: O grams
  - » Sugar: O grams
  - » Cholesterol: O grams
  - » Sodium: O grams
- Potassium: O grams
- Protein: O grams

Remember, everything you do here on your keto diet prepares you for the Mediterranean-keto lifestyle. And trust me when I say it's much easier and more enjoyable! That is where we are going.

If you are one of those who are at or near a healthy weight and want to get straight into the Mediterranean-keto lifestyle (part 2 of this book), that's fine. You will still lose weight, but more slowly and usually not as much as you would on a healthy keto diet. But you will certainly feel better, get healthier, and enjoy the many benefits of the Mediterranean-keto lifestyle. I do recommend to most people, especially if you are trying to lose weight or are fighting a sickness or disease, that you first do the healthy keto diet as we have discussed (part 1).

Then after three to twelve months, after you have experienced ketosis and have a feel for what it's like to live in ketosis, go ahead and shift over to the Mediterranean-keto lifestyle or rotate between the healthy keto diet and the Mediterranean-keto lifestyle.

But as always, it's entirely up to you. This is your life. You get to choose. And because 75 percent of your longevity is a result of the foods you eat rather than the genes you were born with, your choices count.

PART II
THE MEDITERRANEAN-KETO LIFESTYLE

Part 2 explains what the Mediterranean-keto lifestyle is, how it works, the benefits to you, and how to make that lifestyle your own. It is ideally based on someone previously being on a healthy keto diet, but you can jump directly into the Mediterranean-keto lifestyle if you wish. Reading part 1 is still recommended because understanding the ins and outs of a healthy keto diet will help you with your Mediterranean-keto lifestyle.

Chapter 15

A LIFESTYLE WORTH LIVING

MY JOURNEY INTO the Mediterranean-keto lifestyle began with a trip that my wife, Mary, and I took to Greece. A friend of ours grew up in Crete, and she kept telling us about the olive groves, some with trees two thousand years old, and how amazing it was there.

We went during the olive harvest season, and our friend took us to see many things, including her friend's olive press factory, where local farmers would bring their olives to be pressed. There were giant drums that held cold-pressed extra-virgin olive oil that was then bottled and sold locally or exported.

Within an hour of olives going into the press, they would have bottles of fresh olive oil. We were impressed with the process, but there was more to it.

The owner took us into a back room, where he put a couple of shot glasses on a table. Into each he poured about one ounce of the cold-pressed extra-virgin olive oil that had just been pressed.

He told us, "Try it. It's fresh, and it's high in polyphenols, but I'm going to warn you. There will be a tingle in the back of your throat, a mild burning, and a slight cough, but they will go away. With high-quality olive oil you get these symptoms, which are a sign of high-quality olive oil rich in polyphenols."

The tingle is an anti-inflammatory effect. If you have swallowed liquid ibuprofen, you have experienced a very similar feeling. With olive oil, that tingle, burning, and cough is how you know it's high quality.

Mary and I took our little shot glasses of olive oil and tossed them back, swallowing the olive oil in one big gulp. Sure enough, it did burn the backs of our throats. We coughed. But in a flash it was gone. Wow! Never had olive oil caused me such a reaction.

That was my hands-on demonstration of how they screen for high-quality olive oil. Lab tests can also be run on olive oil, checking for polyphenols and oleocanthal. If it doesn't make you cough, if it doesn't burn, then it usually doesn't have the higher concentrations of these powerful polyphenols. It's not bad, of course; it's just that some olive oil is much healthier than already-healthy olive oil.

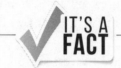

Eating a healthy Mediterranean diet is as or more effective than taking statin medications to reduce cardiovascular events.[1] And there are no side effects!

Believe it or not, there are thirty-six phenolic compounds (polyphenols) in olive oil. These anti-inflammatory compounds protect our arteries against plaque, help the brain, benefit our organs, and so much more. Basically, many of the amazing benefits of a healthy Mediterranean diet are attributed in part or directly to the olive oil.

Across the board, we are not getting enough of the different polyphenols we need. Based on the patients I have had over the past several decades, I would say that very few are getting enough polyphenols on a daily basis. One of the most common polyphenols consumed is chlorogenic acid, from coffee. There are over eight thousand polyphenols found in the foods we eat, such as berries, herbs, spices, veggies, nuts, olives, tea, and cocoa.

One of the many phenolic compounds is oleocanthal, one of the most powerful phytonutrients in the world. It also causes the tingle (and burning and coughing) we experienced. Because oleocanthal is so good for you, it has been highly investigated and researched. It was discovered in 1993, defined in 2005, and found (among many other things) to be like liquid ibuprofen.[2]

POLYPHENOLS

Polyphenols are natural antioxidant compounds that protect us from toxins, prevent blood clots, promote gut health, reduce cell damage, and more. There are two main classes:

1. Flavonoids (60 percent of polyphenols)
2. Phenolic acids (30 percent of polyphenols)

Polyphenols are found in apples, blueberries, blackberries, cranberries, raspberries, strawberries, oranges, grapefruit, lemons, grapes, kiwis, peaches, plums, artichokes, asparagus, broccoli, carrots, cauliflower, spinach, black beans, red/yellow onions, tempeh, tofu, white beans, lentils, almonds, chestnuts, hazelnuts, flaxseeds, pecans, walnuts, ginger, oats, olive oil, rapeseed oil, basil, cinnamon, cloves, cumin, parsley, oregano, rosemary, sage, thyme, black/green/white tea, vinegar, dark chocolate, turmeric, red wine, peppermint, star anise, coffee, black chokeberry, black currants, red currants, capers, black and green olives, hazelnuts, curry powder, celery seed, chicory, shallots, lemon verbena, apricots, caraway seeds, potatoes, endive, nectarines, marjoram, bean sprouts, and red lettuce.[3]

Note: All these foods are living foods, not processed foods.

This oleocanthal is more active than many medications, and it is an anti-inflammatory and a pain reliever. It's also 100 percent natural, which means you get the ibuprofen benefit without any of the side effects.

We've known for decades that olive oil suppresses inflammation, and that inflammation is a root cause of most all chronic diseases, but the fact that high-quality olive oil could also be a pain reliever/painkiller, that was new to me. But that was not all.

ONE SECRET INGREDIENT IN OLIVE OIL: OLEOCANTHAL

Many olive oils have these phenolic compounds but not to the same degree of potency.[4] Oleocanthal, for example, is found in the highest concentrations in extra-virgin olive oil from certain locations in the world. Greece just so happens to be home to several of those locations.

Interestingly, the only known source for this special oleocanthal polyphenol is extra-virgin olive oil. It is found nowhere else. This oleocanthal is actually stronger than ibuprofen as a pain reliever and has been found to help clear beta-amyloid (a sign of Alzheimer's disease) from the brain (benefit 7, chapter 4) and even kill cancer cells.[5] Oleocanthal has been and is being used to fight neurodegenerative diseases, cardiovascular diseases, Alzheimer's disease, cancer (prostate, melanoma, breast, etc.), arthritis, inflammation, and more.[6] (See appendix A, "Recommended Supplements.")

IT'S A FACT

Coffee is the number one source of antioxidants (polyphenol) in the US diet. But if coffee makes you feel sick, wired, tired, as if you can't sleep, or as if your heart has rapid or irregular beats, then don't drink it.[7]

You would think, if extra-virgin olive oil is so good for you and certain areas in Greece boast some of the highest oleocanthal concentrations in the world, that these people would have less sickness and disease and live longer than the rest of us. Well, that is indeed the case.

Back in the 1950s, a physiologist named Ancel Keys from the University of Minnesota did the famous "Seven Countries Study" of diets and habits of people from seven countries (Greece, Italy, Netherlands, former Yugoslavia, Japan, Finland, and the United States). The results: people from Greece lived the longest and had one of the lowest rates of heart disease and consumed the most fat in the form of olive oil.[8]

About ten years ago the small Greek island of Ikaria was reported to have more healthy people over age ninety than anywhere else in the world.[9] It has one of the largest populations of centenarians (people who live to one hundred or more) in the world. Most of this (health, longevity, vitality) I believe is due in part to the incredibly healthy olive oil that is consumed daily.

The full value of oleocanthal to our health and longevity is still being researched, studied, and calculated, but the fact that it's right there in front of us as part of a natural, healthy diet and lifestyle is pretty amazing. It's only one of the great many reasons for choosing to live a Mediterranean-keto lifestyle. Now, we can't all move to Greece or some other Mediterranean country, but thankfully we can all live a healthy Mediterranean-keto lifestyle no matter what city, state, or country we happen to be in.

Chapter 16

SIXTEEN REASONS TO LIVE THE MEDITERRANEAN-KETO LIFESTYLE

A S A MEDICAL doctor, I have always found it satisfying to write a prescription for patients that really works and has no negative side effects! The Mediterranean-keto lifestyle is just that. What's more, anyone can use it. I do primarily recommend it for adults because adults are the ones who usually need it the most, but sometimes it's children.

Not long ago a mom brought her obese eight-year-old son to my office. He also suffered from a fatty liver, which is much more common among adults. In fact, I'd say a third of my adult patients have non-alcoholic fatty liver, but the incidence of younger people having fatty liver is increasing. Today, about 11 percent of adolescents suffer from fatty liver.[1]

A fatty liver is the leading cause of liver disease, but the root of fatty liver is the standard American diet of sugars, carbs, and starches. This boy loved soda, syrup (full of high-fructose corn syrup), honey, pancakes, agave nectar, fruit juices, and the like. Basically, he loved to eat and drink carbs and sugars, and at the age of eight he was already obese. Within three short months on a high-veggie, moderate-protein, low-carb, no-sugar diet that included a lot of olive and avocado oils (simply eating a Mediterranean-keto-style diet), his fatty liver cleared up. He lost weight, his health drastically improved, and the doctor who had been treating him was amazed.

A younger body can usually bounce back more quickly than someone who is older, but it doesn't really matter. You feed your body the right foods and good results are the norm.

That's why a healthy keto diet and the Mediterranean-keto lifestyle are like prescriptions. Children are growing and need more healthy carbohydrates, and that's why I recommend the Mediterranean-keto lifestyle for children and usually start adults with the healthy keto diet. The health changes, benefits, and lives positively impacted are both encouraging and incredible.

THE HEALTH BENEFITS OF THE MEDITERRANEAN DIET

I believe most of the benefits of the Mediterranean diet come from eating more healthy fruits and vegetables; more olive oil; more fish; more beans, peas, and lentils; more nuts and seeds; and some red wine. But equally important is the reduction of red meat, pork, processed meats, processed carbohydrates, starches, and sugary junk foods. In other words, the foods people on a Mediterranean diet don't eat are almost as important as the healthy living foods they do eat.

We have known for many years the tremendous cardiovascular benefits of the Mediterranean diet from several large studies.

The 2003 Lyon Diet Heart Study found that following a Mediterranean diet will reduce the risk of both heart attack and stroke.[2]

- The PREDIMED trial found similar results. The 2003 study divided over seven thousand men and women between the ages of fifty-five and eighty at a high risk for cardiovascular disease into three groups. One group followed a Mediterranean diet but had to consume 1 liter of extra-virgin olive oil each week. A second group followed a Mediterranean diet but also ate at least 1 ounce of nuts a day. A third group ate a low-fat Western diet similar to the American Heart Association's recommended diet.

  The results were astounding. Those in the first two groups, who followed the Mediterranean diet and consumed a liter of olive oil each week or an ounce of nuts a day, saw their risk for all cardiac events and stroke decreased by 30 percent. The results were so dramatic that the study was stopped one year earlier than planned, and the patients on the low-fat Western diet were switched to the Mediterranean diet.[3]

- The 2012 EPIC cohort study of approximately twenty-one thousand people from Greece found that people who followed the Mediterranean diet faithfully and ate the lowest-glycemic foods had the lowest rate of cardio-vascular disease.[4]

New studies also are showing the Mediterranean diet is a protective factor against memory decline and brain atrophy. One German study of individuals at a higher risk of Alzheimer's disease found that those who followed a Mediterranean diet had less memory decline and medial temporal lobe atrophy, which is a biomarker for Alzheimer's disease.[5]

In another study brain-imaging scans were conducted on thirty-plus patients who ate a Mediterranean diet and thirty-plus patients who ate a Western diet. The brain scans were repeated at least two years later. The scans taken at the beginning of the study found that patients who were eating a Western diet already had more deposits of beta-amyloid, a protein that accumulates in the brains of patients with Alzheimer's disease, than those who were eating a Mediterranean diet, and they were only between thirty and sixty years of age. Those who ate a Western diet also had lower energy than those who ate a Mediterranean diet, and this is a sign of lower brain activity. In the follow-up scans two years later, patients on the Western diet showed even more beta-amyloid deposits and a greater reduction in energy, compared with the Mediterranean diet group.[6]

The Mediterranean diet also was shown in the Nurses' Health Study to promote healthy aging. The women who followed a Mediterranean diet were 46 percent more likely to have healthy aging, defined as living to seventy or longer and having no chronic disease or major decline in health.[7] A cohort study from the Nurses' Health Study found that those who followed the Mediterranean diet had longer telomeres. Telomeres are on the ends of DNA, and they shorten with age.

Longer telomeres are considered protective against chronic disease and early death.[8]

These and other studies have shown the tremendous health benefits of the Mediterranean diet; however, I believe there will be even more benefits when the Mediterranean diet is combined with lower-carbohydrate foods.

SIXTEEN REASONS TO ADOPT A MEDITERRANEAN-KETO LIFESTYLE

Here are sixteen very good reasons for living the Mediterranean-keto lifestyle. There are many more, as you will soon find out.

The many health benefits from a healthy keto diet (see chapter 4 for more information) are yours in the Mediterranean-keto lifestyle, but it is important to understand that these benefits are long-term. They are part of the foundation of your healthy lifestyle that you get to live and enjoy for the rest of your life.

If you need to deal immediately with such things as prediabetes, type 2 diabetes, obesity, mild to moderate memory loss, cancers, and other sicknesses and diseases, I usually recommend starting with a healthy keto diet and then shifting over to this Mediterranean-keto lifestyle when the time is right.

Whatever your reason for living the Mediterranean-keto lifestyle, here are sixteen of them, and keep in mind, you get them all:

1. Burns fat instead of sugar—Changing your diet to macronutrient levels as described in the following pages will cause your body to be in and out of ketosis. That means your body will usually burn fat rather than sugar for fuel. Weight loss is the direct result.

2. Snuffs out inflammation—Inflammation is a root cause of virtually every chronic disease (cardiovascular disease, arthritis, most cancers, autoimmune diseases, IBS, psoriasis, most lung disease, Alzheimer's disease, Parkinson's disease, gum disease, depression, autoimmune diseases, etc.), and the Mediterranean-keto

lifestyle helps snuff out inflammation by lowering blood sugar and insulin levels as the foods consumed also decrease inflammation, especially olive oil, fish, veggies, fruits, beans, and red wine.

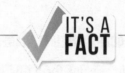

IT'S A FACT

Studies show that coffee may reduce risk of heart disease, dementia, and Parkinson's disease.[8]

3. Provides better blood-sugar control—The Mediterranean-keto lifestyle lowers blood-sugar levels and insulin levels, which help prevent and/or treat type 2 diabetes, prediabetes, and insulin resistance.

4. Helps control appetite hormones—Lower insulin levels from the Mediterranean-keto lifestyle gives you better control of leptin (the appetite hormone).

5. Improves/cures acid reflux—The most common cure of acid reflux is simply losing belly fat and then keeping the weight off, and you get both with the Mediterranean-keto lifestyle.

6. Reduces plaque in arteries—The Mediterranean-keto lifestyle usually lowers blood-sugar levels, blood pressure, and cholesterol levels, and that prevents plaque growth, which is known to lead to heart attacks, strokes, and sudden cardiac deaths. Plaque is usually formed from elevated oxidized LDL cholesterol, elevated blood sugar, and excessive inflammation as well as other factors. The polyphenols, antioxidants, phytonutrients, omega-3 fats, and the Mediterranean-keto lifestyle help quench inflammation in the arteries.

7. Decreases Alzheimer's risk—The Mediterranean-keto lifestyle enables your body to properly regulate insulin levels, and that helps lower the inflammatory proteins, including beta-amyloid, that are directly associated with Alzheimer's disease. The powerful polyphenols, especially oleocanthal, and omega-3 fats are neuroprotective.

8. Lowers triglycerides and usually lowers cholesterol levels—The Mediterranean-keto lifestyle, with its lowered insulin levels and abundance of cholesterol-lowering monounsaturated fats, usually lowers your triglyceride and bad LDL cholesterol levels and usually raises your good HDL cholesterol levels.

9. Prevents and fights cancer—Because cancer cells thrive on sugar, the Mediterranean-keto lifestyle doesn't feed the cancer cells their favorite food. Also, polyphenols, especially oleocanthal, and omega-3 fats support a healthy immune system. I recommend a strict healthy keto diet to fight cancer, but I recommend the Mediterranean-keto lifestyle as the long-term protection against cancer.

10. Helps prevent heart disease—Heart disease is the biggest killer in the world, and the Mediterranean-keto lifestyle helps prevent that by lowering your insulin resistance, reducing your risk of prediabetes and type 2 diabetes, and decreasing inflammation, blood pressure, and cholesterol levels.

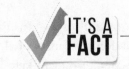

IT'S A
FACT

In 2021 the Mediterranean Diet was rated the best diet overall in the annual best diet ranking for the 4th consecutive year by *US News and World Report*.[10]

11. Decreases arthritis pain—The Mediterranean-keto life-style is anti-inflammatory, and that usually relieves pain for arthritis sufferers.

12. Lowers blood pressure—The Mediterranean-keto life-style usually helps lower blood pressure by lowering insulin levels, which lowers your retention of sodium, and promotes healthy circulation because of the abundance of polyphenols. It also helps one lose belly fat, which also helps to lower blood pressure.

13. Helps a fatty liver—Fatty liver disease (not alcohol related), as we have discussed, can be reversed and protected against with the Mediterranean-keto lifestyle because the healthy fats (e.g., olive oil, which is high in polyphenols) and lowered sugars, carbs, and starches usually improve or reverse a fatty liver when followed for a few months.

14. Improves/cures PCOS—The Mediterranean-keto life-style is ideal for women who suffer from polycystic ovary syndrome (PCOS). The healthy keto diet, followed by the Mediterranean-keto lifestyle, are the best one-two punch for controlling PCOS.

15. Slows down the aging process—The Mediterranean-keto lifestyle lowers sugar levels and helps reduce inflammation in your body, and the foods consumed are usually much higher in antioxidants, phytonutrients, and polyphenols, which in turn slow down the aging process.

16. Prevents most chronic diseases—Insulin resistance and chronic inflammation are causes of almost all chronic diseases, and the Mediterranean-keto lifestyle, with its low-carbohydrate, high-healthy-fat diet, is the best long-term lifestyle answer for insulin resistance and chronic inflammation.

A healthy keto diet is the backbone of the Mediterranean-keto lifestyle, so it only makes sense that you get the same amazing health benefits from a lifestyle as you do from a diet. So whether you begin with a healthy keto diet to meet your specific health goals or you jump directly into the Mediterranean-keto lifestyle as a long-term option, your body benefits.

Imagine being able to stay, day in and day out, in that sweet spot of healthy living where your entire body is happy and healthy! That is what I like about the Mediterranean-keto lifestyle, and that is why I highly recommend it. That's also why I'm living this way myself.

Chapter 17

WHAT THE MEDITERRANEAN-KETO LIFESTYLE LOOKS LIKE

W HEN MARY AND I were in Greece, on the island of Crete, our friend took us out to eat in the evenings. These mom-and-pop restaurants were crowded with locals, and every table had its own bottle of fresh extra-virgin olive oil.

There were six of us at our table, and between us we consumed the entire one-liter bottle of olive oil! But so did everyone else at the other tables. We poured it on the salads, vegetables, soups, meats, breads, and more. Whatever we ate got a liberal dose of olive oil.

The meals were heavy on vegetables and salads (which were often sprinkled with feta cheese), some beans, and fruits, and light on meats (chicken, lamb, fish, etc.). Fresh herbs and spices were plentiful, and all of it was drizzled with olive oil. Of course, there was bread, but very little was eaten.

Produce was fresh, as daily shopping in the open markets was the norm. Homes had small refrigerators because they have no need to store food for long.

At dinner, coffee, tea, and red wine were served. We ate and drank slowly, talking and laughing for two hours—and so did everyone else. It was a much slower pace than we are used to in our eat-on-the-run, eat-in-front-of-the-TV, grab-a-bite-to-eat society, but we loved it (and our stress levels went down).

Not only was everyone freely using olive oil, but the food we ate seemed as if we had planned and then cooked a special meal at home, with fresh low-carb veggies and moderate amounts of healthy proteins, all while being in a restaurant. Without having to do anything, they fed us exactly what the Mediterranean-keto lifestyle looks like.

Earlier (in part 1) I noted that on a pretty strict keto diet, where you are trying to lose weight or overcome a sickness or disease, the food intake usually looks something like this:

- 75 percent fats

- 20 percent proteins

- 5 percent carbs

IT'S A
FACT

The Mediterranean diet was not made by doctors or nutritionists. It's centuries old. It's an eating lifestyle followed by people in southern Europe and northern Africa. It varies, but the core is olive oil, fruits, vegetables, legumes, fish, and wine.

But the more relaxed Mediterranean-keto lifestyle looks like this:

- 50–55 percent fats

- 20–25 percent proteins

- 20–25 percent carbs

What makes the Mediterranean lifestyle keto is that because of the foods the people eat, the olive oil consumption, the salads, the veggies, and the macronutrient proportions, their bodies drift in and out of ketosis. They get the benefits of a healthy keto diet without really having to do anything extra! They don't have to go on a diet like we do, and that's pretty nice. It's their way of life. It's the bottles of extra-virgin olive oil on the tables. It's the healthy, wild, fresh foods. It's the coffee, tea, and red wine. It's the omega-3 and fiber in their foods. It's not eating highly processed foods, not living on a high-sugar and high-carb diet, and not living a sedentary life.

It's a lot of good things, all combined to make their lifestyle, and that is our goal as well. With what you eat in the Mediterranean-keto lifestyle, you will be in ketosis more often than someone who is simply eating Mediterranean foods.

I have found that after your body is used to being in ketosis, you can increase your carbs to around 50–75 grams per day (even 100 grams a day for some) and still be in ketosis. That is another reason for starting with a healthy keto diet before jumping into the Mediterranean-keto lifestyle. But it's always your choice.

TYPICAL MEDITERRANEAN FOODS:

- Olive oil, nuts, and other healthy fats
- Vegetables (fresh salads and sauteed veggies)
- Meats (seafood, poultry, goat, sheep, and cow)
- Fresh herbs
- Beans, peas, lentils, and hummus
- Lower-carb fruits (raspberries, blueberries, black-berries, strawberries, etc.)
- Nuts and seeds
- Yogurt and kefir
- Eggs
- Dark chocolate
- Coffee, black tea, and water
- Red wine (in moderation: one glass per day, or best, not at all)

If your starting point is the Mediterranean-keto lifestyle, then 50 grams of carbs per day is recommended, especially for the first few months while your body is adapting to burning fat for fuel rather than burning sugar for fuel. Then you can slowly increase to 75–100 grams of carbs per day, and eventually up to 125 grams of carbs per day for some. That is still much fewer carbs than the typical American consumes, which is 250–500 grams of carbs a day.

THE BASICS OF THE MEDITERRANEAN-KETO LIFESTYLE

A typical Mediterranean diet is higher in carbs than what we are describing here on the Mediterranean-keto lifestyle. That simply means that you can't and don't want to eat everything you find labeled Mediterranean.

It's the same with keto diets. Some are not as healthy as others. What you want to do, and what we are doing here, is select the healthy foods that accomplish your healthy goals and eat those foods in the proper proportions.

At a glance, the Mediterranean-keto lifestyle is going to include basics, such as

- healthy fats

- healthy proteins

- eating a lot of vegetables and salads

- eating moderate amounts of proteins

- eating low-to-moderate amounts of healthy carbs, usually ½ cup with 2–3 meals, and best as beans, peas, or lentils (pressure-cooked) and low-carb fruits.

This lifestyle avoids or minimizes

- packaged foods (cereals, cookies, pizza)

- processed foods (bacon, sausage, granola, crackers, chips)

- dairy (milk, cheese, ice cream), except for small amounts of feta cheese

- fake sugars and sweets

- high-carb, high-sugar foods

- unhealthy fats (margarine, shortening, excessive saturated fats, fried foods, and soybean, corn, and canola
  oils).

What does that look like in real foods? In the back of the book are recipes for the Mediterranean-keto lifestyle, but how that looks is different per person. It is, after all, your lifestyle.

As you know, the Mediterranean-keto lifestyle is based on these macronutrient levels:

- 50–55 percent fats

- 20–25 percent proteins

- 20–25 percent carbs

That is the new norm. At times, that may fluctuate a bit, but that's the framework on which you can base your food and health decisions.

IT'S A FACT

The number one cause of heart disease is not high cholesterol. Rather, it's elevated blood-sugar levels from eating too much sugar and refined carbs.[1]

How that breaks down depends on your own numbers, your health goals, and whether you are trying to lose or maintain your weight. (If you are fighting a sickness or disease, or need to lose a lot of weight, then I suggest starting with a healthy keto diet as explained in part 1.)

Perhaps you are looking at the 50–55 percent fats, 20–25 percent proteins, and 20–25 percent carbs and wondering how you could eat so much or so little of these each day. If so, then you may need to pause. Flip back to chapters 8, 9, and 10. They explain the details behind each of these important macronutrients.

A healthy Mediterranean diet that is also low in sugars and carbs, as we describe here, is incredibly healthy. Eating that way has a proven track record that will encourage and perhaps even amaze you. Here is another quick snapshot of how it looks:

- decreased incidence of dementia

- improved kidney function

- lowered rates for type 2 diabetes

- reduced depression

- improved bone density

- reduced risk of some cancers

- weight loss

- reduced risk of heart disease

- 50 percent of deaths associated with cardiovascular disease eliminated[2]

As you know, olive oil is an integral part of the Mediterranean-keto lifestyle, just as it is with a healthy keto diet. What is interesting as well as comforting is that Mediterranean food and olive oil have a direct correlation with lower cancer rates.[3] In fact, for over twenty years, nineteen different studies tracked more than thirty-five thousand people and found that olive oil use was directly linked to lower cancer risks.[4] And for women specifically, those who stuck with a Mediterranean diet and all of its extra-virgin olive oil had a much lower level of breast cancer risk than the normal population.[5]

Beans, peas, and lentils are also a very important component of the Mediterranean-keto lifestyle (in moderation) if you have no gut issues. They are packed with protein, vitamins, minerals, and fiber and help control blood sugar while blocking disease-causing oxidation.[6] They also have some starch (which counts as a sugar) and lectins, which are inflammatory compounds.[7] But removing the lectins is easy enough. Simply soak the beans overnight in water with a little salt and discard the water the next morning. Then you pressure-cook them for at least seven and a half minutes. The soaking and cooking process removes almost all the lectins, thereby decreasing inflammation.

Here are several different beans and their macronutrient details for a half cup:

- black—7 grams fiber, 8 grams protein, 20 grams carbs, 13 grams net carbs

- green snap—1.9 grams fiber, 1.9 grams sugar, 1.4 grams protein, 3.7 grams carbs, 1.8 grams net carbs

- pinto—7.5 grams fiber, 7.5 grams protein, 22.5 grams carbs, 15 grams net carbs

- red kidney—7 grams fiber, 2 grams sugar, 7 grams protein, 19 grams carbs, 12 grams net carbs

- fava—4.5 grams fiber, 6.5 grams protein, 16.5 grams carbs, 12 grams net carbs

- garbanzo—6 grams fiber, 7.5 grams protein, 22.5 grams carbs, 16.5 grams net carbs

- lima—4.5 grams fiber, 6 grams protein, 20 grams carbs, 15.5 grams net carbs

- navy—9.5 grams fiber, 0.3 grams sugar, 7.5 grams protein, 23.5 grams carbs, 14 grams net carbs

- white—5.5 grams fiber, 8.5 grams protein, 22 grams carbs, 16.5 grams net carbs

- lupini—2.3 grams fiber, 13 grams protein, 7.5 grams carbs. 5.2 grams net carbs

Other healthy carbs include, but are not limited to, such foods as sweet potatoes, yams, cassava, and taro root, usually limited to the size of a tennis ball, or half a cup per serving.

If you want a lifestyle that keeps you healthy, charges your metabolism so you can lose weight, and helps protect you from countless sicknesses and diseases, I cannot recommend anything better than the Mediterranean-keto lifestyle. That is where we are headed.

THE DANGER OF LECTINS

Lectins are large proteins found in plants and concentrated in the leaves and seeds of all plants but are also found in animals that eat these plants. Lectins are concentrated in grain, especially wheat, but also in legumes (beans, including soybeans, peas, and lentils) as well as nightshades (plants such as tomatoes, potatoes, peppers, and eggplant).

Lectins may and usually eventually do trigger inflammation in the gut and may trigger inflammation in the entire body. They bind to sugar molecules (sialic acid) found in the gut, joints, and brain as well as other locations and may cause inflammation, brain fog, joint pain, and gut issues, to name a few. Lectins also usually cause weight gain.[8]

Corn and brown rice also contain lectins, though white rice has significantly fewer lectins. A particularly nasty lectin that causes weight gain is wheat germ agglutinin (WGA) found in wheat bran. WGA is found in whole wheat products, including whole wheat bread and whole wheat pasta. WGA behaves similarly to insulin, causing weight gain, and may eventually lead to the development of insulin resistance.

Today's wheat is potentially very inflammatory for many of my patients. Wheat can produce 23,788 different proteins,[9] and any of these have the potential of triggering inflammation. However, most inflammation from wheat is caused by two specific gluten proteins: glutenin and gliadin.

The typical Mediterranean diet contains a lot of wheat products as well as other inflammatory carbs. For this reason, I recommend low-lectin carbs in moderation and low-carb fruits, 50–100 grams per day. If you have gut issues, please read my book *Healthy Gut Zone* before starting the Mediterranean-keto lifestyle.

Farmers have known for many years that pigs and cattle are fattened up mainly by eating corn and soy beans and not by eating grass or hay. Wheat, corn, and soy are all loaded with lectins and are in most processed foods.

On the Mediterranean-keto lifestyle, we need to avoid most of these high-lectin foods and starches and choose beans, peas, or lentils that have been soaked and pressure-cooked for seven and a half minutes to remove most of the lectins. Other low-lectin carbs include sweet potatoes, yams, cassava, jicama, taro root, yucca, and millet bread.

The approximate numbers will help you:

- ½ cup beans typically contains about 10–20 grams net carbs

- a medium sweet potato contains 27 grams carbs

- a single slice of millet bread contains 11 grams carbs

- 1 cup jicama contains 12 grams carbs

- 1 cup taro root contains 23 grams carbs

- ½ cup cassava contains 39 grams carbs (limit and minimize)

- ½ cup basmati white rice contains 36 grams carbs (limit and minimize)

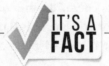

IT'S A
FACT

Even though apples are considered a higher-carb fruit, I still recommend one apple a day because of the following benefits.

- Helps control one's weight. The soluble fiber (pectin) in apples is filling and reduces one's appetite, which helps to control one's weight.

- Boosts the immune system. Red apples contain the powerful antioxidant quercetin, which boosts immune function. That is the reason doctors have been saying for decades, "An apple a day keeps the doctor away."

• Helps reduce cholesterol and blood sugar. The soluble fiber (pectin) in apples helps reduce cholesterol levels and control blood sugar, preventing or curbing blood-sugar swings.

• Helps prevent gallstones and hemorrhoids. The soluble fiber in apples helps lower cholesterol, which is what most gallstones are composed of, thereby preventing gallstones. The fiber also supports regular bowel movements and helps prevent straining, which prevents hemorrhoids.[10]

One or two servings a day of low-carb fruits are also good to add to your Mediterranean-keto lifestyle. You do not have to choose a starch with each meal. A starch at dinner is what I usually do since it helps me sleep and maintain my weight. Many people, however, prefer to have a single fruit serving with two meals a day on the Mediterranean-keto lifestyle and one starch a day once they have reached their weight goal.

Here are some low-carb fruits:

• raspberries (½ cup): 7.5 grams carbs

• blackberries (½ cup): 7 grams carbs

• lemon (1 whole): 7.8 grams carbs

• strawberries (½ cup): 5.5 grams carbs

• lime (1 whole): 7.1 grams carbs

• plum (1 medium): 7.5 grams carbs

• clementine (1 medium): 8.9 grams carbs

• kiwi (1 medium): 10 grams carbs

• blueberries (½ cup): 9.7 grams carbs

• cantaloupe (½ cup): 7 grams carbs

- watermelon (½ cup chopped): 6 grams carbs

Here are some higher-carb fruits:

- apple (1 medium): 25 grams carbs

- pear (1 medium): 27 grams carbs

- peach (1 large): 17 grams carbs

- pineapple (1 cup): 22 grams carbs

- mango (1 medium): 50 grams carbs

- grapes (1 cup): 16 grams carbs

- banana (1 medium): 27 grams carbs

Dried fruit, such as figs, prunes, raisins, and cranberries, are especially high in carbs. The USDA recommends that the average adult consume two cups of fruit a day, but stick with the low-carb fruits to keep your weight in check.

Chapter 18

THREE STEPS TO STARTING YOUR MEDITERRANEAN-KETO LIFESTYLE

WHEN YOU ARE ready to jump into your Mediterranean-keto lifestyle, there are a few steps that you need to take first. If you have been on a healthy keto diet, this will probably be second nature for you.

Also, if you are coming to the Mediterranean-keto lifestyle after being on a healthy keto diet, then adding more carbs (in the form of beans, peas, lentils, hummus, sweet potatoes, low-sugar fruits, and other healthy carbs) will most likely be a welcome change.

Any journey starts by first knowing both where you are and where you are going. With the Mediterranean-keto lifestyle, that means knowing what types of foods and how much of these healthy foods you should be eating every day. That is simple enough.

Here are the three steps that everyone starting the Mediterranean-keto lifestyle needs to take:

STEP 1: ESTIMATE YOUR CALORIES

Begin by calculating your calories based on the Mediterranean-keto lifestyle macro levels: 50–55 percent fats, 20–25 percent proteins, and 20–25 percent carbs.

How that looks will vary between men and women, but it can also vary from person to person. Each of our bodies is different, so the following breakdown is an average fits-most-people set of numbers. If your body requires more or less of something, you will probably know as you grow more accustomed to your body's needs and your ever-improving health.

For women

The average adult woman in the United States consumes around 1,600–2,400 calories in food per day. To lose weight, you want to decrease that to 1,600 calories per day while maintaining these Mediterranean-keto lifestyle macro numbers.

Based on calories per day, that means

- 800 calories from fats

- 400 calories from proteins

- 400 calories from carbs.

- 1 gram of fat = 9 calories
- 1 gram of carb = 4 calories
- 1 gram of protein = 4 calories

For men

The average adult male in the United States consumes around 2,400–3,800 calories in food per day. To lose weight, you should decrease your food intake to 2,400 calories per day while maintaining these Mediterranean-keto lifestyle macro numbers.

Based on 2,400 calories per day, that means

- 1,200 calories from fats

- 600 calories from proteins

- 600 calories from carbs.

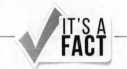

7 grams of protein = 1 ounce (e.g., 4 ounces of fish = 28 grams of protein)

STEP 2: ESTIMATE YOUR GRAMS

Once you know your calories per macronutrient level, you can convert that to grams. According to the USDA, the calories-to-grams ratio for fats is 9 calories per 1 gram of fat, 4 calories per 1 gram of protein, and 4 calories per 1 gram of carbs.

For women at 1,600 calories per day, that would be about

- 89 grams fats (6.6 tablespoons fats per day)
- 100 grams proteins (14.3 ounces proteins per day)
- 100 grams carbs.

For men at 2,400 calories per day, that would be about

- 133 grams fats (10 tablespoons fats per day)
- 150 grams proteins (21.4 ounces proteins per day)
- 150 grams carbs.

For both men and women who are trying to lose weight or want to hold their weight where it is, they will probably want to lower the carbs a little. I suggest 75 grams for women and 100 grams for men. That is usually sufficient for gradual weight loss for most people.

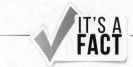

Olive oil is incredibly healthy, and you will learn to like its taste in time. However, don't use it in smoothies. Use avocado, almond, or macadamia oils in smoothies, as these cold-pressed oils have very little taste. I also sometimes use macadamia nut oil in my coffee with chocolate collagen. It gives it a buttery taste and lowers cholesterol levels.

Also, the lower the carb level is, the longer your body will stay in ketosis, and that is where fat burning takes place.

If you are jumping into the Mediterranean-keto lifestyle directly, you will want to track your daily caloric intake as you get started so you know you are right on target while you are getting used to eating a set number of calories/grams per day. It also helps as you plan, consider recipes, and choose your meals, and that is probably going to feel like the most important part of your journey.

STEP 3: ESTIMATE YOUR GRAMS PER MEAL

For women eating 1,600 calories over three meals per day, the macronutrient breakdown is approximately

- 30 grams fats per meal (2.2 tablespoons per meal)

- 33 grams proteins per meal (4.8 ounces per meal)

- 33 grams carbs per meal. (I recommend 25 grams per meal initially to lose weight and then slightly more carbs to maintain weight.)

For men eating 2,400 calories over three meals per day, the macronutrient breakdown is approximately

- 44 grams fats per meal (3.3 tablespoons per meal)

- 50 grams proteins per meal (7.1 ounces per meal)

- 50 grams carbs per meal. (I recommend 33 grams or less per meal initially to lose weight and then slightly more carbs to maintain weight.)

Now that you know the macronutrient amounts required for the necessary fats, proteins, and carbs of your Mediterranean-keto lifestyle, you are ready to begin. Thankfully, all of the math and calculations per macro and recipes have already been figured out. You don't have to do it all!

You can easily find out (from books, online, apps, etc.) what the macronutrients are per food item, and what's more, you don't have to build your entire recipe list on your own (unless you want to). Use the many recipes in the back of this book to begin, but there are hundreds more to choose from online.

Chapter 19

TEN TIPS FOR YOUR MEDITERRANEAN-KETO LIFESTYLE

T HE MEDITERRANEAN-KETO LIFESTYLE is just that—a lifestyle. It will eventually come naturally to you, from food choices to amounts to recipes to buying food, so don't put pressure on yourself to know everything or do everything just right.

Practice this. Take your time. Learn as you go. Metaphorically speaking, it's like learning to ride a bike. You can do it with no hands later on but not today.

As you launch into your Mediterranean-keto lifestyle, here are ten tips that will make the launching process easier, quicker, and more hassle-free:

TIP 1: REMEMBER WHY YOU ARE HERE

Always remember your goals and why you are here. Besides eating healthier foods (honestly, almost anything is better than the standard American diet), what motivates you to want to live a healthier lifestyle? Is there a family history of sickness or disease that you are trying to avoid? I find that to be very common with many of my patients, and it is a strong motivation to choose foods wisely and take care of our bodies.

Or perhaps it's to lose weight? To enjoy the kids, grandkids, and great-grandkids? To keep up with your spouse? So you can travel more? Or to simply live the life you've always wanted?

Whatever motivated you to start this Mediterranean-keto lifestyle, keep it in the forefront of your mind. It's not that the Mediterranean-keto lifestyle is hard or arduous; it's just always good to remember why you are here.

TIP 2: KEEP MEAL PLANNING SIMPLE TO START

The best way to keep meal planning simple in the beginning is to use the already-created Mediterranean-keto lifestyle recipes found in the back of this book. Start there. It's easy. It's simple. You don't have to think or plan, and that's very helpful.

Later you can begin to widen your reach, look for other recipes, experiment, have fun, and try new things. And as long as it fits within the healthy macronutrient parameters (50–55 percent fats, 20–25 percent proteins, 20–25 percent carbs), then you are on target.

TIP 3: PLAN EACH WEEK IN ADVANCE

At this point, while you are getting used to the foods and macronutrient amounts and olive oil and all the other details in your new Mediterranean-keto lifestyle, it's best to set your week's menu. Then simply follow it. By planning ahead for each week, it will make your shopping so much easier. You also won't have to think very much about it. And as you get into the flow of things, this is very important.

I suggest planning a week in advance for at least your first month and maybe even your first three months. Many people make this their habitual practice. It's up to you, but when you are starting, don't make yourself think too hard.

TIP 4: RESTOCK AS NEEDED

You will quickly find that many of the foods in your fridge or pantry are not viable options in your new Mediterranean-keto lifestyle. You may grab a sauce or syrup or juice (typical high-sugar-content items) out of habit, but when you read the ingredients, you will most likely see that there are too many carbs in it.

Maintaining your macronutrient levels (50–55 percent healthy fats, 20–25 percent healthy proteins, 20–25 percent healthy carbs) to fit your Mediterranean-keto lifestyle is the answer to pretty much all foods in question. When in doubt, simply ask yourself, "Does this food/drink fit my Mediterranean-keto lifestyle?"

If not, don't eat or drink it. But if you do eat or drink something that isn't part of your plan, such as at holidays, when you are a guest, on special occasions, or for some other reason, don't feel bad or pressure yourself. It's certainly not the end of the world. Tomorrow is a new day. (I will often chase those types of foods down with 1 tablespoon of psyllium husk powder, which can bind to it and help clear it out.)

In your own home and with your usual routine, you will need to restock your fridge and pantry. I suggest to most people that they do this in the beginning when they start their healthy keto diet or Mediterranean-keto lifestyle. An extra benefit of clearing things out is that it also removes any temptation to eat comfort foods along the way.

If you first did the healthy keto diet and you put the beans, peas, and lentils on the back of the shelf, you can get them out now. I enjoy beans, and they are a vital part of Mediterranean fare.

Use this list to help you restock your fridge and pantry:

- oils—olive and avocado especially (in dark glass containers), MCT oil (powder or liquid), coconut, almond, walnut, macadamia

- vegetables—avocado, arugula, cabbage, cucumbers, broccoli, celery, spinach, kale, chard, seaweed, romaine, artichokes, bean sprouts, green beans, Brussels sprouts, olives, radish, cauliflower, greens (collard, mustard, dandelion), asparagus, garlic, mushrooms, onions (of all sorts), summer squashes (yellow squash, zucchini), spaghetti squash, peppers, eggplant, and tomatoes

- low-sugar fruits—strawberries, raspberries, blackberries, blueberries, limes, lemons, plums, clementines, kiwi, cantaloupe, watermelon

- eggs (organic and/or free-range)

- fresh/dried herbs—ginger, oregano, basil, cilantro, parsley, thyme, rosemary, sage, mint, bay leaves, chili powder, cumin, curry powder, paprika, black pepper, dillweed, cayenne pepper, red pepper flakes, cinnamon, cardamom, etc.

- nuts/seeds—almonds, walnuts, Brazil nuts, peanuts, pecans, macadamias, cashews, hazelnuts, pine nuts, pistachios, chia, flax, hemp, poppy, pumpkin, safflower, sesame, sunflower, etc.

- pickled/fermented foods—kefir (especially goat and sheep), dill pickles, kimchi, sauerkraut, miso, apple cider vinegar, banana peppers, capers, olives, pickled jalapeños, etc.

- condiments—mustard, avocado mayo, pesto sauce, low- or no-sugar hot sauces, sugar-free ketchup, marinara sauce, vanilla extract, tomato paste, red wine vinegar, balsamic vinegar

- meats—pasture-raised poultry (including turkey) and eggs; wild or sustainably harvested fish, oysters, wild smoked salmon, tongol tuna, etc.; grass-fed beef, bison, pork, sheep, goat, etc.; wild deer, rabbit, elk, etc.

- dairy (to be limited to less than 10 percent of your total daily fat intake)—feta, grass-fed ghee, grass-fed butter, sour cream, heavy whipping cream, cheese, cream cheese, unsweetened yogurt, almond milk, coconut milk

- broths—chicken, beef, bone

- natural sweeteners—stevia, monk fruit, erythritol

- coffee, tea, and water (filtered)

- fiber (psyllium husk powder)

- dark chocolate (70 percent or higher cacao)

- healthy carbs to be added in the Mediterranean-keto lifestyle—beans (black, green, snap, pinto, red, kidney, garbanzo, lima, navy, white, lupini), lentils, peas (green and black-eyed), sweet potatoes, yams, cassava, taro root, gluten-free bread or gluten-free pasta, basmati white rice, millet bread, low-sugar fruits, and other healthy carbs

- supplements (See appendix A, "Recommended Supplements.")

TIP 5: TRACK UNTIL YOU WANT TO QUIT TRACKING

When you first start your Mediterranean-keto lifestyle, you will need to carefully track the calories and grams of the fats, proteins, and carbs you eat. It's simply necessary when you start. Eating prescribed recipes will certainly help in that regard, especially if you don't like tracking.

But the good news (for most people) is that once you feel your Mediterranean-keto lifestyle has become a habit, you can pretty much quick tracking your daily intake. I strongly recommend that you track your macronutrient levels for your foods for the first month and ideally for the first three months if you can. After that, you will have a basic feel for what fits the Mediterranean-keto lifestyle and what does not.

TIP 6: BE PATIENT WITH YOURSELF

Do be patient with yourself. The Mediterranean-keto lifestyle is worth your time and effort, but it's a lifestyle, which is long-term thinking. So be nice to yourself. Be patient. And don't worry, you will get the hang of all this eventually.

You will even be able to cook your own Mediterranean-keto lifestyle foods spontaneously! Yes, it will happen, so be patient with yourself while you are learning.

TIP 7: EXERCISE REGULARLY

Exercise is a vital part of the Mediterranean-keto lifestyle. Even if you are only walking twenty to thirty minutes a day, three to five days a week, that is a good place to start. Make it your habit to be up, active, and mobile.

Though weight loss usually increases with more exercise, being active is vital to good heart health, clear thinking, energy levels, healthy gut, good mood, and so much more. My suggestion is to make a habit of twenty to thirty minutes of walking or exercise of some sort (aerobics, weights, bicycling, etc.) at least three to five times a week. Let that be your goal and eventual new baseline. Then when you want or need to do more, your body can handle it. This is, after all, a lifestyle.

TIP 8: YOU ALWAYS CALL THE SHOTS

You are the one who is responsible to figure out what's best for you. This is *your* Mediterranean-keto lifestyle after all. With the macronutrient levels of 50–55 percent fat, 20–25 percent protein, and 20–25 percent carbs, there is some fluctuation. I have had patients who range from 40–60 percent with fats, 20–30 percent with proteins, and 10–25 percent with carbs. (Those with an intense daily workout routine can usually do 25 percent carbs and still be in and out of ketosis).

It is a combination of these macronutrients that enables your body to be in ketosis and burn fat for fuel. The usual cause for being bumped out of ketosis is too many carbs. Occasionally it's from too much protein (excess protein is converted to sugars in the body), but I have never seen it from too many healthy fats.

So it's your carb percentage that you need to monitor the most. It's your own individual percentage. For me, I can have a little gluten-free bread or some beans at night (carbs help you sleep) but not too much. Around 75 grams of carbs total in one day is good for me. That maintains my weight, keeps my brain sharp, and fuels my workouts, and I slip in and out of ketosis most days. If I really need to focus at work, then I'll decrease my carbs that day. I find around 30–50 grams of carbs gives me greater mental clarity, and I also increase my fats on those days.

For you and your body, your carb percentage may be higher or lower. For most people, I suggest they keep it around 75–100 grams per day, but it's up to you to find and maintain.

TIP 9: REMEMBER THE BASICS

Here is a quick checklist of basics that we all need to keep in mind as we live the Mediterranean-keto lifestyle:

- Go with the flow—We can't avoid carbs for the rest of our lives. The answer is to rotate carbs. Some days you will have more; some you will have less. Cycle back and forth, keeping your macronutrient levels always in mind, and your body will overall be able to maintain its healthy state.

- Watch your carbs—This is the most common cause for bumping you out of ketosis (the fat-burning state). It may be from eating too much food, drinking too much alcohol, carbs/sugars/starches in foods, hidden sugars, or another source.

- Watch your saturated fat intake—As with the healthy keto diet, try to keep saturated fats to 10 percent or less of your daily intake. Our bodies need some saturated fat, but too much causes inflammation.

- Get sufficient fiber—Fiber is found in vegetables, nuts, fruits, beans/peas/lentils, and psyllium husk powder (a supplement). You need 30–35 grams of fiber per day, but start low and go slow.

- Get sufficient omega-3 (fish oil)—I suggest 1,000 milligrams per day from supplements (as close to a 2:1 ratio EPA:DHA as you can). Let what you get from foods (e.g., wild-caught fish) be extra.

- Mind the APOE4 gene—Drinking red wine is a regular part of every Mediterranean culture, and a little red wine is actually good for the brain *if* you do not have the APOE4 gene. (See chapter 6 for more information.) If you have memory problems or early dementia, get the APOE gene test right away. If you don't have it, a little red wine (one 4-ounce glass a day) is OK. I do, however, recommend that you avoid alcohol entirely or until you have taken an APOE gene test and gotten the results back.

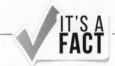

Consuming fiber, regardless of your age, is a necessity. It

- helps control appetite and cravings
- helps control blood-sugar and insulin levels
- decreases inflammation
- lowers blood pressure
- improves cholesterol
- helps remove toxins from your body
- prevents constipation
- feeds healthy bacteria in your gut.[1]

TIP 10: ENJOY YOUR NEW LIFESTYLE

As they say, "Slow down and smell the roses." That's good advice, especially as it applies to your Mediterranean-keto lifestyle. Enjoying life is actually good for your health!

This applies especially to meal times. Eat more slowly. Chew each bite at least twenty times. Talk and laugh. Don't watch the news, argue, or rehash stresses from work while eating. Relax so that your body can better digest your food.

Overall, learn to worry less. Find ways to destress yourself. Play games, tickle your grandchildren, listen to calming music, read books, take dance lessons, go for walks, sit and watch the sun go down, have tea with a friend, tend your garden, and get a good night's sleep. A lifestyle is meant to be enjoyed.

Chapter 20

GO AHEAD, TASTE YOUR MEDITERRANEAN-KETO LIFESTYLE

Looking at the Mediterranean-keto lifestyle, there is no question as to its health value, both for the now and for the future. So what's next?

Tasting the food! The recipes in the following pages need to be tested and tasted to be believed. This is no dry, packaged meal plan. Rather, this is fresh, vibrant, colorful, healthy, and delicious! If you are ready to jump into the Mediterranean-keto lifestyle, then I suggest that you simply spend your next week eating the foods that are listed in part 3. I'm guessing you will not only enjoy them, but you may notice a few health benefits in that short amount of time.

Our bodies are designed to self-heal, and when we feed our bodies the right foods, the results can sometimes be amazing. In as little as a few weeks, I have seen improvement and even complete reversal in many of my patients with such things as

- headaches
- acid reflux
- brain fog
- weight gain
- food cravings
- aching joints
- high blood-sugar levels
- muscle pain

- fatigue

- insomnia

- high insulin levels

- nasal congestion

- memory problems

- constipation

- IBS

- high blood pressure

- and more.

If any of these describe you, trust me when I say that this is just getting started. You have already seen the many health benefits of the Mediterranean-keto lifestyle. They are yours, ready and waiting. And they can be yours for the rest of your life. That is what I love!

So go ahead. Jump in. Your Mediterranean-keto lifestyle awaits.

PART III

RECIPES FOR A HEALTHY MEDITERRANEAN-KETO LIFESTYLE

Part 3 includes delicious recipes for a healthy Mediterranean-keto lifestyle with swaps you can make if you're following a strictly keto diet. These recipes are ideal for starting out, and you can repeat them as many times as you want, but soon you will want to gather your own recipes that meet your individual macronutrient needs. Begin with these recipes, and enjoy. Thankfully food can taste great and help you achieve your health goals.

Chapter 21

TASTY MEAL IDEAS

THE MEDITERRANEAN-KETO LIFESTYLE enables you to keep off weight and avoid sickness and disease. These benefits can be the foundation of a healthy lifestyle that you get to enjoy for the rest of your life. The core of this lifestyle is healthy fats (e.g., olive oil, avocado oil, nut oils), fruits, a lot of non-starchy vegetables, small to moderate amounts of legumes, nuts, moderate amounts of lean meats and fish, and occasional wine, but this lifestyle is still low in sugars and carbs.

The Mediterranean-keto recipes in the following meal plan incorporate more carbs than a strictly keto diet and follow these macro levels: 50–55 percent fats, 20–25 percent proteins, and 20–25 percent carbs. Many people find 75–100 grams of net carbs to be their sweet spot for maintenance. Keep in mind that higher-carb foods such as rice, gluten-free pasta, sweet potatoes, and cassava should still be occasional foods a few times a week, though a serving of legumes each day is OK. As I mentioned previously, it's best to use dry legumes, soak them overnight, and pressure-cook them to remove inflammatory lectins. Then add them to a recipe or as a side.

If you want or need to go through a keto diet for weight loss before switching to the more relaxed Mediterranean-keto lifestyle, look for the "strictly keto" modifications noted with some recipes. To lose weight, women shouldn't exceed 1,600 calories per day and men shouldn't exceed 2,000 to 2,400 calories per day. That amounts to roughly 450 to 600 calories per meal for women and approximately 600 to 800 calories per meal for men. Men can increase their portions or add more oil to their meals to increase their caloric intake.

Again, remember your macros. Keep your net carbs at 20 grams a day to stay in ketosis (fat-burning mode) and aim for 75 percent fats, 5 percent carbs, and 20 percent proteins.

For women at 1,600 calories eating three meals per day, that means approximately

- 44 grams of fats per meal (around 3.33 tablespoons of fats per meal)

- 27 grams of proteins per meal (around 4 ounces of proteins per meal)

- 7 grams of carbs per meal.

For men at 2,400 calories eating three meals per day, that means approximately

- 67 grams of fats per meal (around 5 tablespoons of fats per meal)

- 40 grams of proteins per meal (around 6 ounces of proteins per meal)

- 10 grams of carbs per meal (or 7 grams per meal if you choose 20 grams of carbs per day).

If you are starting at a different number of calories per day, divide your daily calorie goal by your intended number of meals per day, and keep each meal within that range. As usual on a keto diet, watch the carbs from fruits, higher-carb nuts and vegetables, starches, and beans. As I mentioned, I have found that after their bodies get used to being in ketosis, many people can increase their net carbs to around 50–75 grams per day and will still be in ketosis—some can go as high as 100 grams per day.

If your starting point is the Mediterranean-keto lifestyle, then 50 grams of carbs per day is recommended to begin as your body gets used to burning fat instead of sugar for fuel. Then you can slowly increase to 75–100 grams of carbs per day. Some can go as high as 125 grams of carbs per day and maintain a healthy weight. If you find yourself gaining weight, reduce the amount of carbs you're eating each day.

Mix and match the following meal ideas until you get familiar with the types and amounts of foods to eat on a daily basis. Then, after you have practiced with these recipes for a few weeks, begin to seek out other recipes or experiment with your own. I believe you'll find, as I did, that a Mediterranean-keto diet isn't just healthy; it's delicious.

BREAKFASTS

Breakfast Scramble

1 teaspoon grass-fed ghee

3 tablespoons avocado oil, divided

½ cup yams, diced

¼ cup broccoli, chopped

¼ cup onions, chopped

¼ cup button mushrooms, sliced

¼ cup spinach, shredded

2 organic pasture-raised eggs

1 link cooked chicken sausage or 2–3 slices of turkey or regular bacon (nitrate/nitrite-free), diced

¼ cup berries

Heat ghee and 1 tablespoon of avocado oil over medium heat. Add the yams. Cook 3–4 minutes. Add veggies and cook 3–4 minutes more, until tender. In a small bowl, whisk eggs. Add to veggies and stir until desired doneness. Top with diced meat of your choice. Drizzle with remaining avocado oil. Serve with a side of berries. (1 serving)

Mediterranean-keto:

Calories: 567; net carbs: 27 grams

Strictly keto: Women use 2 eggs, men use 3 eggs, and omit the yams and berries.

Calories (2 eggs): 458; net carbs: 5 grams
Calories (3 eggs): 529; net carbs: 5 grams

Fruit and Almond Pancakes

Fruit Syrup:

½ cup strawberries

½ cup chopped peaches

2 tablespoons avocado oil

2 tablespoons grass-fed ghee

½ teaspoon debittered stevia (optional)

Pancakes:

4 large eggs

½ cup almond flour

1 tablespoon stevia (debittered)

¼ teaspoon baking powder

¼ cup avocado oil

¼ cup sliced or slivered almonds

Coconut cream (optional)

Organic natural almond or peanut butter (optional)

Cook strawberries, peaches, avocado oil, and ghee over low heat until fruit is soft. Stir in stevia and let cool. In a small bowl, whisk eggs. In a separate bowl, combine almond flour, stevia, and baking powder. Stir half of the avocado oil into the eggs. Whisk dry ingredients into egg mixture. Use remaining avocado oil to grease a griddle or frying pan. Heat over medium-low heat. Ladle ¼ cup of batter onto pan. Sprinkle almonds on top of each pancake. Flip pancakes after 2–3 minutes, when edges are no longer moist. Top with fruit syrup. If desired, add a dollop of coconut cream sweetened with stevia (50 calories; 1 gram of net carbs per tablespoon), or spread natural almond butter (98 calories; 1 gram of net carbs per tablespoon) or peanut butter (94 calories; 2 grams of net carbs per tablespoon) on pancakes before topping with syrup. Makes 6 pancakes.

Mediterranean-keto:

Syrup—calories per tablespoon: 68; net carbs: 1.5 grams

Pancakes (each, without coconut cream or nut butter)—calories: 186; net carbs: 2 grams

Strictly keto: Omit the peaches from the syrup and use 1 cup strawberries. If you choose to top pancakes with nut butter, use almond butter instead of peanut butter. Suggested serving: 2 pancakes for women (372 calories; 4 grams net carbs) with 2 tablespoons syrup (135 calories; 2 grams net carbs) and 3 pancakes for men (558 calories; 6 grams net carbs) with 3 tablespoons syrup (203 calories; 3 grams net carbs).

Syrup—calories per tablespoon: 68; net carbs: 1 gram

Chocolate Peanut Butter Shake

1 cup unsweetened almond or coconut milk

½–1 teaspoon dark unsweetened cocoa powder

¼–½ teaspoon stevia (debittered)

1 tablespoon avocado or macadamia nut oil (2 tablespoons for men)

2 tablespoons organic peanut butter or almond butter

1 scoop Keto Zone chocolate hydrolyzed collagen protein powder

½ cup ice

Place all the ingredients in a blender and process until smooth. (1 serving)

Mediterranean-keto:

Calories: 437; net carbs: 5 grams

Men (with extra tablespoon avocado or macadamia nut oil)— calories: 557; net carbs: 5 grams

Strictly keto: Use almond butter.

Calories: 445; net carbs: 4 grams

Men (with extra tablespoon avocado or macadamia nut oil)— calories: 565; net carbs: 4 grams

Nutty Cereal

3 cups unsweetened shaved coconut

1 cup finely chopped walnuts, pecans, and almonds

1 tablespoon coconut oil, melted

1 tablespoon macadamia nut oil, melted

1 tablespoon vanilla extract

½ teaspoon stevia (debittered)

1 tablespoon cinnamon

½ teaspoon sea salt

Preheat oven to 300 degrees. In bowl, mix coconut and nuts. In separate bowl, whisk oil, vanilla, stevia, and cinnamon. Drizzle over nut mixture and stir well. Spread mixture onto lined baking sheet. Bake until lightly toasted, stirring occasionally. Remove from oven and cool. Makes 4 cups. Recommended serving: ⅔ cup for women and 1 cup for men served with an equal amount of unsweetened almond, coconut, or oat milk.

Mediterranean-keto:

2/3 cup without milk—calories: 377; net carbs: 6 grams

1 cup without milk—calories: 566; net carbs: 9 grams

Strictly keto: Serve with almond milk (30–40 calories; 1 gram net carbs per cup).

Salmon and Avocado Lettuce Wraps

2–4 butter lettuce leaves

1 medium avocado, cut into wedges

2–4 tomato slices

2–4 onion slices

6–8 ounces smoked salmon slices (my favorite is Biltmore wild Alaskan sockeye salmon)

Lemon wedges

Himalayan salt

White or black sesame seeds

Place tomato and onion slices in bottom of each butter lettuce leaf. Layer smoked salmon on top. Add 2 avocado wedges to each wrap and mash down slightly with a fork. Sprinkle with lemon juice, salt, and sesame seeds. Suggested portion size: 6 ounces salmon for women and 8 ounces salmon for men. (1 serving)

Mediterranean-keto:

8 ounces salmon—calories: 541; net carbs: 7 grams

6 ounces salmon—calories: 421; net carbs: 6 grams

Strictly keto: No modifications needed.

Keto Breakfast Porridge

2 tablespoons ground flaxseed

2 tablespoons ground chia seeds

2 tablespoons unsweetened shredded coconut

1–2 teaspoons granulated sweetener of choice (erythritol, monk fruit, debittered stevia)

½ cup hot unsweetened oat, almond, or coconut milk

½–1 cup cold unsweetened oat, almond, or coconut milk

3 tablespoons chopped nuts (hazelnuts, walnuts, almonds, pecans)

¼ cup raspberries, strawberries, blueberries, or blackberries

Dash of cinnamon or nutmeg (optional)

Splash of vanilla extract (optional)

Combine dry ingredients in a small bowl. Add the hot liquid and stir well. It will be thick! Add the cold liquid, stirring until desired consistency, similar to oatmeal. Stir in nuts, berries, and spices. To prepare the night before, add an extra 4 tablespoons of liquid to thin mixture. Place it in fridge. (1 serving)

Mediterranean-keto:

Calories: 458; net carbs: 6 grams

Strictly keto: Use coconut or almond milk.

Quick Berry Muffin

3 tablespoons almond flour

1 tablespoon coconut flour

1 tablespoon erythritol or ½ teaspoon stevia (debittered)

¼ teaspoon baking powder

Pinch of salt

1 large egg

1 teaspoon grass-fed ghee (melted and cooled)

2 tablespoons avocado oil (3 tablespoons for men.)

¼ teaspoon vanilla extract

8 blueberries or raspberries

Whisk the flours, sweetener, baking powder, and salt in a large microwave-safe mug. In a separate small bowl, whisk the egg, ghee, oil, and vanilla. Mix into the dry ingredients. Gently stir in the blueberries. Smooth the top of the batter.

Place mug in the microwave for 1 minute 15 seconds. If the muffin is not cooked through, cook 15 seconds more. Carefully remove the hot mug from the microwave. Flip it upside down over a plate. Spread with ghee if desired. (1 serving)

Mediterranean-keto:

Calories (with 2 tablespoons avocado oil): 492; net carbs: 6 grams

Calories (with 3 tablespoons avocado oil): 612; net carbs: 6 grams

Strictly keto: No modifications needed.

Berry Power Smoothie

1 cup unsweetened almond or coconut milk, or more as needed

¼ cup frozen or fresh blueberries, raspberries, or strawberries

¼ cup clementine segments or fresh plums

2 tablespoons unsweetened cashew butter

1 tablespoon ground flaxseed or chia seeds

1 tablespoon avocado oil

1 scoop Keto Zone vanilla hydrolyzed collagen powder

1–2 teaspoons stevia (debittered) or monk fruit sweetener (optional)

Splash of vanilla extract (optional)

Dash of ground cinnamon (optional)

Place all ingredients in a blender and process until smooth and creamy, adding more almond milk as needed to achieve your desired consistency. (1 serving)

Mediterranean-keto:

Calories: 487; net carbs: 19 grams

Strictly keto: Use macadamia nut butter or almond butter in place of cashew butter. Do not add clementine segments or plums.

Calories: 452; net carbs: 7 grams

Green Deviled Eggs

4 large hard-boiled eggs

2 tablespoons lemon juice

1–2 tablespoons extra-virgin olive oil

1 clove garlic, minced

1 red chili pepper, seeded and minced

1 avocado, chopped

Salt and pepper to taste

4 slices cooked turkey bacon or bacon, crumbled

1 tablespoon minced fresh chives

Halve eggs lengthwise. Gently scoop out the yolks and mash them with the avocado. Mix in the lemon juice, olive oil, garlic, chili pepper, salt, and pepper. Spoon the mixture back into the egg white halves. Top with bacon and chives, and serve chilled. Makes 8 deviled eggs. Suggested serving: 4 deviled eggs for women, 6 deviled eggs for men.

Mediterranean-keto:

Each deviled egg—calories: 99; net carbs: 1 gram

Strictly keto: No modifications needed.

Hearty Vegetable Frittata

2 large eggs (3 for men)

1 tablespoon fresh chopped or ½ teaspoon dried herbs, such as rosemary, thyme, oregano, basil

Salt and pepper to taste

1 tablespoon avocado oil

1 tablespoon extra-virgin olive oil (2 tablespoons for men)

½ cup chopped fresh spinach, arugula, kale, or other leafy greens

2 ounces artichoke hearts, quartered, rinsed, drained, and dried

4 cherry tomatoes, cut in half

1 tablespoon diced black or Kalamata olives

¼ cup crumbled soft goat or feta cheese

Preheat the oven to broil on low. Whisk eggs, herbs, salt, and pepper in a small bowl. Heat avocado oil over medium heat in a small oven-safe skillet or omelet pan. Add the spinach, artichoke hearts, and cherry tomatoes, and sauté 1–2 minutes. Add the egg mixture and let it cook undisturbed over medium heat for 3 to 4 minutes, until bottom begins to set. Sprinkle the olives and cheese on the egg mixture. Transfer the skillet to the oven to broil for 4–5 minutes, or until the frittata is firm in the center and golden on top. Remove from the oven. With a spatula, loosen the frittata from the sides of the pan. Gently flip it onto a plate or platter. Drizzle with the olive oil. (1 serving)

Mediterranean-keto:

2 eggs with 1 tablespoon olive oil—calories: 511; net carbs: 5 grams

3 eggs with 2 tablespoons olive oil—calories: 702; net carbs: 5 grams

Strictly keto: No modifications needed.

Keto Zone Coffee

6–8 ounces brewed hot coffee

1 tablespoon MCT oil powder

¼–½ teaspoon stevia (debittered)

1 tablespoon macadamia nut oil (optional, for buttery, nutty flavor)

½–1 teaspoon dark unsweetened cocoa powder (optional)

1 scoop Keto Zone chocolate hydrolyzed collagen (optional)

Place all the ingredients in a blender and process until smooth and foamy. Or briskly stir the oil, stevia, and cocoa powder into hot coffee. (1 serving)

Mediterranean-keto:

Calories: 271; net carbs: 0 grams

Strictly keto: No modifications needed.

LUNCHES

Avocado and Tomato Salad

2 tablespoons extra-virgin olive oil

1 teaspoon lemon juice (or to taste)

1 clove garlic, minced

¼ cup basil, torn

1 avocado, chopped

½ cup chopped tomato

1 tablespoon walnuts or pecans, chopped

Salt and pepper to taste

1 ½ cups fresh spinach or greens

Whisk oil, lemon, and garlic. In a separate bowl, combine basil, avocado, tomato, and walnuts. Toss with oil mixture. Season with salt and pepper. If you'd like to add protein, toss in chunks of cooked fish, shrimp, chicken, or steak. Serve over greens. (1 serving)

Mediterranean-keto:

Calories: 545; net carbs: 7 grams

Strictly keto: No modifications needed, but women will need to add minimal (1–2 ounces) or no protein to keep from exceeding the recommended calories per meal.

Garlicky Shrimp and Asian Cucumbers

Shrimp:

2 tablespoons sesame oil

1 tablespoon reduced-sodium, gluten-free soy or tamari sauce or liquid aminos (such as Bragg's)

4 cloves garlic, minced

1 teaspoon arrowroot powder

1 tablespoon fish sauce (optional)

2 tablespoons avocado oil

1 pound wild raw shrimp, peeled and deveined, tails on

2 green onions, minced

Asian Cucumber Salad:

2 cups sliced cucumbers

¼ cup sliced sweet onions

½ cup cooked green peas

2 tablespoons sesame oil

1 tablespoon apple cider vinegar

2 teaspoons sesame seeds

1 garlic clove, minced

Salt and pepper to taste

Whisk sesame oil, soy sauce, garlic, arrowroot, and fish sauce until smooth. Set aside. Heat avocado oil over medium heat. Add shrimp and cook for 1–2 minutes per side. Pour sauce over shrimp. Simmer for 5 minutes. Top with green onions. Separately mix salad ingredients together. Serve shrimp with ¼ cup of cooked white basmati rice (51 calories; 11 grams net carbs) or quinoa (56 calories; 9 grams net carbs) and 1 cup salad. (2 servings)

Mediterranean-keto:

Shrimp dish without sides (6 ounces)—calories: 474; net carbs: 4 grams

Salad (1 cup)—calories: 194; net carbs: 9 grams

Strictly keto: Omit peas from side salad. Serve shrimp without rice or quinoa. To stay within optimal calorie range, women have 4 ounces of shrimp and men have 6–8 ounces of shrimp.

Shrimp dish (4 ounces)—calories: 316; net carbs: 2 grams

Salad (1 cup)—calories: 163; net carbs: 3 grams

Chili-Spiced Salmon Over Wilted Spinach

Salmon:

3 to 6 ounces wild salmon

1 tablespoon extra-virgin olive oil

¼ teaspoon garlic powder or to taste

¼ teaspoon chili powder or to taste

Salt and pepper to taste

Juice of ½ lemon

Spinach:

1 tablespoon grass-fed ghee

1 10-ounce bag baby spinach

1 garlic clove, minced

2 tablespoons extra-virgin olive oil

Juice of ½ lemon

Salt and pepper to taste

¼ cup gluten-free pasta (optional)

Brush salmon with olive oil. Sprinkle with garlic powder, chili powder, salt, and pepper. Grill over medium heat until fish flakes easily with fork. Remove from heat, and drizzle with lemon juice and olive oil.

Heat ghee in a large skillet over low heat. Add the spinach and cook until just wilted. Add the garlic, salt, and pepper, and cook 1 minute. Remove from heat. Drizzle with olive oil and lemon.

Break up salmon into bite-size pieces. Toss with spinach and serve with ¼ cup of gluten-free garbanzo/chickpea pasta if desired. Sprinkle with extra lemon juice, olive oil, salt, and pepper as needed. (1 serving)

Mediterranean-keto:

Calories (with 6 ounces salmon): 781; net carbs: 6 grams (Add 190 calories and 24 grams net carbs if you serve with gluten-free chickpea pasta, such as the Banza brand.)

Strictly keto: Omit the gluten-free pasta; serve salmon over the spinach. I recommend women have 3 ounces of salmon and drizzle only 1 tablespoon of olive oil over spinach. This will result in 540 calories and 6 grams of net carbs.

Seeded Bread Sandwiches

Bread:

3 tablespoons ground chia seeds

3 tablespoons ground psyllium seeds

¾ cup raw sunflower seeds

¾ cup ground flaxseeds

1 cup ground hemp seeds

¾ cup ground pumpkin seeds

1 teaspoon salt

½ teaspoon stevia (1 packet)

1½ cups water

1½ tablespoons avocado oil

1½ tablespoons grass-fed ghee, melted

Sandwich fillings:

Nitrate-/nitrite-free ham or turkey

Avocado wedges

Sliced tomato

Sliced cucumber

Hummus

Feta cheese

Avocado oil mayonnaise

Yellow or stone-ground mustard

Combine seeds, salt, and stevia in a large bowl. In a separate bowl, whisk together the water, oil, and ghee. Pour the liquid mixture into the seed mixture. Mix well. Let stand for 2 to 3 hours. Preheat the oven to 350. Line a loaf pan with parchment paper. Pour batter into the pan, and bake 70–80 minutes. Cool completely, then slice for sandwiches. Makes 10 slices. (10 servings)

Build sandwiches with fillings of choice, staying mindful of your macros. Serve sandwich with a side of guacamole and a few (four or five) cassava chips.

Mediterranean-keto:

Calories per slice: 298; net carbs: 0.5 grams

Nitrate/nitrite-free ham or turkey (60–70 calories; 2 grams net carbs per ounce); ¼ avocado (80 calories; 1 gram net carbs); sliced tomato (5 calories; 1 gram net carbs); sliced cucumber (5 calories; 1 gram net carbs); hummus (80 calories; 2 grams net carbs per 2 tablespoons); feta cheese (70 calories; 1 gram net carbs per ¼ cup); avocado oil mayonnaise (90–100 calories; 0 grams net carbs per tablespoon); yellow or stone-ground mustard (4 calories; 0 grams net carbs per tablespoon); guacamole (70 calories; 1 gram net carbs per 2 ounces)

Strictly keto: Serve guacamole with celery or jicama slices (49 calories; 5 grams net carbs per cup) instead of cassava chips. Make sure sandwich fillings don't exceed 200 calories. Women, use 1 slice of bread and make sandwich open-faced to keep calories between 450 and 600.

Keto Burgers and Sweet Potato Wedges

2 sweet potatoes, cut into wedges

1 tablespoon avocado or coconut oil

Salt and pepper

1 pound grass-fed ground beef

2 teaspoons garlic powder

1 teaspoon salt

½ teaspoon pepper

½ cup feta cheese

Romaine or butter lettuce

Tomato slices (optional)

Onion slices (optional)

Avocado slices (optional)

Mustard (optional)

Avocado oil mayo (optional)

Preheat oven to 400. Drizzle sweet potato wedges with avocado oil and season with salt and pepper. Bake for 15–20 minutes. While potatoes bake, add garlic powder, salt, and pepper to ground beef. Mix well then shape into 4 patties. Grill or broil the burger to desired doneness. When you flip the burgers, top each burger with feta cheese. Serve burgers between 2–4 lettuce leaves, topped with tomato, onion, mustard, mayo, and avocado. (4 servings)

Mediterranean-keto:

With sweet potato wedges but without burger toppings—calories: 413; net carbs: 14 grams

Strictly keto: Omit the sweet potato wedges. Instead, serve with a side salad made with 1 cup lettuce, ½ avocado, 1 tablespoon olive oil, 1 teaspoon vinegar, and lemon juice to taste (241 calories; 2 grams net carbs) or a side salad made with lettuce, tomato, cucumbers, 1 tablespoon olive oil, and 1 teaspoon vinegar (145 calories; 4 grams net carbs). Men may add another 2 tablespoons olive oil to add 240 calories.

Burger without toppings or side salad—calories: 325; net carbs: 2 grams

Cilantro Chicken Soup

1 (3–4 pound) free-range chicken, skin removed; 14 ounces frozen grilled chicken fajita strips; or whole rotisserie chicken

Organic chicken broth (enough to cover chicken, 1–2 quarts)

Himalayan salt to taste

1 cup onions, chopped

1 cup mushrooms, chopped

1 cup broccoli, chopped

¼–½ cup peppers (optional)

¼–½ cup fresh cilantro, chopped

6–8 tablespoons extra-virgin olive oil or avocado oil

½–1 cup white basmati rice, cooked

Place the chicken, enough broth to cover chicken, and salt in a slow cooker. Cook on low for 3–4 hours. (To save cooking time, you can also cook the chicken in a stockpot on the stove. Bring to a boil, reduce to a simmer, and cook for 1 hour 15 minutes. Then reduce heat to low.) Remove chicken from the cooker or pot and let sit until cool enough to handle. Pull chicken from bones in bite-size pieces. Return chicken meat to cooker or pot. Add vegetables, cilantro, olive oil, and rice 15 to 30 minutes before serving so they don't get too soft. Ladle soup into bowls in 1½-cup portions. (4 servings)

For a faster soup, use a rotisserie chicken and remove skin and pull meat off bones in bite-size pieces, or use frozen grilled chicken fajita strips. Put meat in pot on stovetop with enough broth to cover the chicken. Bring to a boil, then simmer for 20 to 30 minutes. Add veggies, cilantro, olive oil, and rice, and simmer until veggies are softened. If desired, serve with a side salad made with 1 cup lettuce, 4 slices tomato, 1 tablespoon olive oil, 1 teaspoon apple cider vinegar, salt, pepper, and lemon juice to taste (195 calories; 3 grams net carbs).

Mediterranean-keto:

1 ½ **cups**—calories: 549; net carbs: 18 grams

Strictly keto: Omit rice. Men add 1–2 tablespoons olive oil to add another 120–240 calories.

1 ½ **cups**—calories: 489; net carbs: 5 grams

Chicken or Tongol Tuna Salad on Greens

Salad:

3–4 tablespoons avocado oil mayo

¼ cup chopped celery

¼ cup chopped onions

3–6 ounces cooked chopped chicken or (low-mercury) tongol tuna[*]

Celery seed, celery salt, garlic or garlic salt (optional)

Salt and pepper to taste

* Tongol tuna, which can be found at health-food stores, is very low in mercury.

Any mix of butter lettuce, arugula, field greens, or spinach

¼ cup sliced cucumbers

¼ cup sliced tomatoes

½ cup white or garbanzo beans

1 tablespoon sunflower seeds

¼ cup feta or soft goat cheese, crumbled

Oil and Vinegar Dressing

¼ cup apple cider vinegar

¾ cup extra-virgin olive oil or avocado oil

Onion juice to taste

Minced garlic or garlic powder to taste

Dried oregano to taste

Salt and pepper to taste

Combine mayo, celery, onion, chicken/tuna, salt, pepper, and spices. Mix well. Fill salad bowl with greens. Top with vegetables, beans, then chicken/tuna salad. Whisk dressing ingredients together, and drizzle a few tablespoons over salad. Sprinkle with feta or goat cheese. You also may substitute butter lettuce for greens and put chicken/tuna salad between 2 butter lettuce leaves and eat as a sandwich. (1 serving)

Mediterranean-keto:

Salad with 6 ounces meat—calories: 644; net carbs: 20 grams

Dressing per 2 tablespoons—calories: 180; net carbs: 0 grams

Strictly keto: Omit beans from salad recipe. I recommend 3 ounces chicken or tuna for women and 6 ounces for men.

Salad with 3 ounces meat—calories: 397; net carbs: 7 grams

Salad with 6 ounces meat—calories: 540; net carbs: 7 grams

Keto-Friendly Chili

2 pounds grass-fed ground beef

2 tablespoons avocado oil

1 medium yellow onion, chopped

3 to 4 cloves garlic, minced

1 tablespoon tomato paste

2 tablespoons chili powder

2 teaspoons ground cumin

1 can (14-ounce) diced tomatoes

⅓ cup water

1 can (14-ounce) black, pinto, or kidney beans

1 green bell pepper, diced (optional)

Sliced green onions (optional)

Sliced jalapeños (optional)

Cilantro (optional)

In a large pot, brown the ground beef. Drain the meat, reserving half of the drippings. Set aside meat. Add oil to drippings and heat pan. If desired, add bell pepper, onion, and garlic, and cook until lightly browned. Stir in tomato paste, chili powder, and cumin. Cook for 1 minute. Add water, tomatoes, and ground beef. Stir to combine. Bring to boil, then lower heat to a gentle simmer and cook for 1-2 hours. (Alternatively: After browning meat, transfer to a slow cooker and add remaining ingredients, except beans and toppings. Cook 4-6 hours.) Add beans and warm through. Top with green onions, jalapeños, and cilantro as desired. (6 servings)

Mediterranean-keto:

1 cup—calories: 518; net carbs: 14 grams

Strictly keto: Omit beans. I recommend men add 1 or 2 tablespoons avocado oil or a green salad with tomatoes, onions, and Oil and Vinegar Dressing to increase calories.

1 cup—calories: 460; net carbs: 7 grams

Fajita Skewers

1 pound grass-fed steak, cut in cubes

1 tablespoon chili powder

1½ teaspoons paprika

1 teaspoon ground cumin

½ teaspoon garlic powder

½ teaspoon salt

¼ cup avocado oil

Juice of 2 limes

1 large onion

1 green or red bell pepper

15–20 mushrooms

6 skewers

Place the cubed steak in a large container and set aside. Cut onion and pepper into 1-inch chunks. Add onion, pepper, and mushrooms to container with steak.

In a small bowl, combine the spices, salt, oil and lime juice. Whisk well, and pour into the container with steak and veggies. Place lid on container, and gently shake to distribute marinade. Place in the refrigerator for 30 to 45 minutes, shaking container 2 times while marinating.

Preheat a grill to medium-high heat. Thread roughly 3 ounces of steak, along with peppers, onions, and mushrooms onto the skewers. Grill the kabobs for 7 to 10 minutes, turning halfway, until desired doneness on steak. Makes 6 skewers.

May eat with a salad made with 1 cup of romaine lettuce, ¼ cup each of tomatoes, onions, and cucumbers, and a simple dressing made with 2 tablespoons of extra-virgin olive oil and 2 teaspoons of vinegar. (277 calories; 6 grams net carbs)

Mediterranean-keto:

1 skewer—calories: 201; net carbs: 5 grams

Strictly keto: Omit one vegetable to reduce carbs. Suggested serving: 2 skewers for women and 3 for men.

1 skewer—calories: 191; net carbs: 3 grams

Keto Cobb Salad

3 cups mixed greens

3–6 ounces cooked pasture-raised chicken or turkey

1 slice cooked bacon or turkey bacon, diced

1 large egg, hard-boiled and sliced

4 grape tomatoes, halved

½ avocado, sliced or cubed

¼ cup sliced mushrooms

2 tablespoons low-carb ranch dressing (made with avocado or extra-virgin olive oil such as Primal Kitchen's ranch dressing)

¼ cup soft goat or feta cheese crumbles (optional)

Place greens in a large bowl. Add bacon, egg, tomatoes, avocado, onion, and mushrooms. Top with dressing and cheese. (1 serving)

Mediterranean-keto:

With cheese and 6 ounces chicken or turkey—calories: 747; net carbs: 7 grams

Strictly keto: No modifications needed, but I recommend women use 3 ounces meat and ½ ounce cheese to remain within their calorie limits.

With 2 tablespoons cheese and 3 ounces chicken or turkey—calories: 560; net carbs: 7 grams

DINNERS

Asian Stir Fry

1½ tablespoons avocado oil

1½ tablespoons sesame seed oil

3–6 ounces chicken cut into bite-size pieces

2 cups veggies (broccoli, cabbage, bok choy, green onion, peppers, mushrooms)

1 garlic clove, minced

½ tablespoon fresh ginger, minced

1 teaspoon organic soy sauce (gluten-free, non-GMO) or tamari sauce

Chili garlic sauce to taste

Sesame seeds

1 green onion, minced

¼ cup cooked basmati rice

Heat the avocado and sesame seed oils in a large skillet over medium heat. Add the chicken, turning after 3–4 minutes. Cook until almost done. Add vegetables, garlic, and ginger and cook until tender-crisp, stirring occasionally. Remove from heat. Drizzle with avocado oil and gluten-free soy sauce. Dot with chili garlic sauce for spiciness. Sprinkle with sesame seeds and green onion. (1 serving)

Mediterranean-keto:

With 6 ounces chicken—calories: 860; net carbs: 33 grams

Strictly keto: Omit rice. Women use 3 ounces of chicken and 1 tablespoon each of the sesame seed and avocado oils to stay within their calorie limits. Men use 6 ounces of chicken.

With 3 ounces chicken, 1 tablespoon sesame seed oil, and 1 tablespoon avocado oil—calories: 515; net carbs: 7 grams

With 6 ounces chicken—calories: 741; net carbs: 7 grams

Shrimp Scampi

1 tablespoon grass-fed ghee

4 tablespoons avocado oil, divided

4–8 ounces raw wild shrimp, peeled

1 clove garlic, minced

Juice of ½ lemon

2 tablespoons dry white wine

Salt and pepper to taste

1–2 cups asparagus or broccoli

Heat the ghee and 3 tablespoons avocado oil in a skillet over medium heat. When melted, add the shrimp. Turn shrimp once, and cook until pink throughout, about 3 minutes. Add the garlic, lemon, wine, salt, and pepper. Cook 1 minute. Remove from pan. Heat remaining oil. Sauté asparagus or broccoli for 3–4 minutes. Season with salt and pepper. (1 serving)

Mediterranean-keto:

With 8 ounces shrimp—calories: 875; net carbs: 7 grams

Strictly keto: Omit wine from sauce and use no more than 1½ cups of veggies. Women use 4 ounces of shrimp and cook it in 1 tablespoon of ghee and 2 tablespoons of avocado oil. Men use 8 ounces of shrimp and cook it in 1 tablespoon of ghee and 3 tablespoons of avocado oil.

With modifications for women—calories: 497; net carbs: 6 grams

With modifications for men—calories: 717; net carbs: 6 grams

Mediterranean-Keto Pizza

Crust:

¼ cup coconut flour, sifted

¼ teaspoon salt

½ teaspoon herbs and spices (any mixture of basil, thyme, garlic powder, oregano, red pepper flakes, etc.)

2 tablespoons ground psyllium husks

1 tablespoon avocado or extra-virgin olive oil

1 cup warm water (not boiling)

Sauce:

1/2 cup low-sugar tomato sauce

1 teaspoon herbs and spices (basil, thyme, garlic powder, oregano, red pepper flakes)

1 tablespoon extra-virgin olive oil

Toppings:

Olives

Nitrate/nitrite-free sliced ham or cooked chicken strips

Artichoke hearts

Roasted red peppers

Mushrooms

Onions

½ cup goat cheese or feta crumbles or part-skim mozzarella cheese

¼ cup pine nuts, toasted

Fresh herbs (basil, oregano, thyme)

Preheat the oven to 400°F. Line a large baking sheet with parchment paper. In a large mixing bowl, combine coconut flour, salt, herbs/spices, psyllium husks, oil, and water. Mix well then knead the dough for 2 to 3 minutes. The batter may seem a little wet, but that's OK. Set dough aside for 15 minutes. Meanwhile, combine tomato sauce, herbs/spices, and 1 tablespoon olive oil. Sprinkle coconut or almond flour on counter or rolling sheet. Roll the dough out to ½-inch thickness. Place on baking sheet. Top crust with tomato sauce and toppings of choice. Bake for 12 to 15 minutes, or until the edges of the crust are slightly brown. Garnish with toasted pine nuts and fresh herbs. (2 servings)

Mediterranean-keto:

½ **pizza**—calories: 599; net carbs: 14 grams

Strictly keto: Omit pine nuts and use smaller amounts of the veggies. If desired, add a green side salad made with 1 cup lettuce, ½ avocado, 1 tablespoon olive oil, 1 teaspoon vinegar, and lemon juice to taste (241 calories; 2 grams net carbs) or with spinach, goat or feta cheese, 1 tablespoon olive oil, and 1 teaspoon vinegar (165 calories; 1 gram net carbs). Men add 1 more ounce feta or goat cheese (75–80 calories; 1–2 grams net carbs per ounce) and/or 1–2 tablespoons olive oil (120–240 calories) if needed to increase calories.

½ **pizza**—calories: 375; net carbs: 7 grams

Tip: This pizza has a few extra carbs, so lower the carbs on your other meals to account for them. If you don't want to make your own pizza crust, buy a low-carb cauliflower-crust pizza. There are several brands that are very low in net carbs. For instance, the Cali'flour brand's traditional flavor has 90 calories and 1 gram of net carbs per serving. (If you have a hard time digesting cauliflower, take an alpha-galactosidase enzyme product such as Beano before you eat to prevent stomach upset.) I like to put olive oil on the crust, then pizza sauce, then goat or part-skim mozzarella cheese. Then I add toppings: lots of mushrooms and onions, a small amount of ham, then a little minced garlic on top. That makes a delicious pizza!

Chinese Chicken Strips

1/3 cup quinoa

1 cup coconut milk

1 cup water

Cilantro to taste

Green onions, sliced

4 tablespoons organic gluten-free soy sauce (non-GMO)

4 tablespoons rice vinegar

1/2 teaspoon sesame oil

1 teaspoon red pepper flakes

4 tablespoons chicken broth

½ teaspoon ground ginger

½ teaspoon onion powder

6 boneless skinless chicken breasts, cut into strips

2 eggs

1 cup almond flour

3 tablespoons avocado oil

Cook quinoa according to package instructions, using coconut milk for half of the liquid and water for the remaining half. When quinoa is ready, stir in cilantro and green onions. Serve in ¼-cup portions.

To prepare the meat, whisk soy, vinegar, ½ teaspoon of sesame oil, red pepper flakes, chicken broth, ginger, and onion powder in a bowl. Add chicken and marinate for 30 minutes up to 2 hours. In a separate bowl, whisk the eggs. Pour the almond flour onto a shallow plate. Drain marinade. Dip chicken pieces into the almond flour, coating all sides, and then dip it into the egg mixture. Heat avocado oil in large pan over medium heat. Cook chicken for 7–8 minutes, turning strips halfway, until brown and cooked through. Garnish with green onions. Serve with quinoa and a side of sautéed vegetables such as cabbage or broccoli. (4–6 servings)

Mediterranean-keto:

With 6 ounces chicken—calories: 761; net carbs: 15 grams

Strictly keto: Omit quinoa. Increase amount of sautéed vegetables on the side to 1 cup. Suggested serving: 4 ounces chicken for women and 6 ounces for men.

With 4 ounces chicken—calories: 491; net carbs: 6 grams

With 6 ounces chicken—calories: 652; net carbs: 6 grams

Curried Shrimp and Broccoli

1 tablespoon avocado oil

1 tablespoon extra-virgin coconut oil

1 pound raw wild shrimp, peeled

1 tablespoon yellow curry powder

¼ teaspoon cinnamon

Salt and pepper to taste

2 oranges, seeded and quartered

½ cup snap peas, cut in half

Fresh cilantro

1 tablespoon extra-virgin olive oil

2 cups broccoli, chopped

Salt and pepper to taste

Lemon wedges

Heat avocado and coconut oils in a skillet over medium heat. Add shrimp and cook for about 2 minutes per side. Add curry powder, cinnamon, salt, pepper, orange pieces, and peas, stirring well. Cook until shrimp are pink and start to curl and oranges are browned. Garnish with fresh cilantro before serving.

In a separate pan, heat olive oil and cook broccoli until tender, stirring occasionally. Season with salt, pepper, and lemon juice. (2 servings)

Mediterranean-keto:

With 6 ounces curried shrimp—calories: 498; net carbs: 20 grams

Strictly keto: Omit snap peas and oranges. Add 1 cup cabbage sautéed in 1 tablespoon olive oil (132 calories; 1.6 grams net carbs). Men can cook 2 cups veggies in 2 tablespoons olive oil to add 264 calories and 3.2 grams net carbs.

With 6 ounces curried shrimp—calories: 433; net carbs: 5 grams

Stuffed Pork Chops

1 slice cooked bacon, diced

½ cup chopped white mushrooms

2 ounces goat cheese, crumbled

1 teaspoon chopped fresh rosemary

1 large clove garlic, minced

2 (12-ounce) bone-in pork chops (about 1 inch thick)

½ teaspoon salt

¼ teaspoon pepper

¼ teaspoon garlic powder

1 tablespoon avocado oil

Preheat the oven to 350. In a small bowl mix bacon, mushrooms, goat cheese, rosemary, and garlic. Cut a large slit in the side of each pork chop. Do not cut all the way through. Stuff the pork chops with the mushroom filling, then press closed and secure with toothpicks or twine. Season the chops with salt, pepper, and garlic.

Heat the avocado oil in an oven-safe pan over medium-high heat. Sear each side of the pork chops, about 2 to 3 minutes per side. Transfer the pan to the oven and bake for 25 to 30 minutes. Internal meat temperature should reach 145. Allow the pork chops to rest for 3 to 5 minutes before serving. Serve with ½ cup roasted yams and a side salad made with lettuce, tomato, cucumbers, 1 tablespoon olive oil, and 1 teaspoon vinegar. (2 servings)

Mediterranean-keto:

Including yams and salad—calories: 788; net carbs: 20 grams

Strictly Keto: Suggested serving: 8 ounces of pork for women and 12 ounces for men. Omit yams. Serve with a salad made with 2 cups lettuce, ½ cup tomatoes, ½ cup cucumbers, 2 tablespoons olive oil, and 2 teaspoons vinegar (279 calories; 5 grams net carbs) and/or 1 cup green beans sautéed in 2 tablespoons olive oil (271 calories; 4 grams net carbs). Men may add 1–2 tablespoons olive oil if needed to increase calories.

6 ounces pork—calories: 281; net carbs: 1 gram

8 ounces pork—calories: 375; net carbs: 1 gram

Garlic Steak and Cauliflower Rice

2 grass-fed rib eye steaks, 3 ounces each

1 tablespoons grass-fed ghee, divided

1 tablespoon avocado oil, divided

2 cloves garlic, minced

1 medium head cauliflower

2 tablespoons extra-virgin olive oil

1 clove garlic, minced

Salt and pepper

Grill or pan sear rib eyes over medium heat until desired doneness. In a small pan, melt the ghee; then add the garlic and avocado oil. Cook for 1 minute. Drizzle ghee and avocado oil over top of steaks.

Core the cauliflower and chop coarsely. Pulse cauliflower in food processor until it looks like large pieces of rice. In a large skillet over medium heat, heat the olive oil. Add the garlic and sauté for 1 minute. Add the riced cauliflower and cook for about 10 minutes or until the cauliflower rice is tender. Season with salt and pepper. (2 servings)

Mediterranean-keto:

6 ounces steak and 2 cups cauliflower rice—calories: 501; net carbs: 10 grams

Strictly keto: Limit cauliflower rice to 1 cup. Add green salad made with 1 cup lettuce, ½ avocado, 1 tablespoon olive oil, 1 teaspoon vinegar, and lemon juice to taste. Suggested serving: 4 ounces steak for women and 6 ounces for men.

4 ounces steak with cauliflower rice and salad—calories: 542; net carbs: 7 grams

6 ounces steak with cauliflower rice and salad—calories: 644; net carbs: 7 grams

Macadamia Nut–Crusted Wild Tilapia

2 (4-ounce) wild tilapia fillets

½ cup unsalted macadamia nuts

1 tablespoon chopped fresh parsley

1 tablespoon fresh lemon juice

2 tablespoons avocado oil

¼ teaspoon garlic powder

Salt and pepper to taste

2 tablespoons olive oil

Lemon wedges, for serving

Preheat the oven to 400 degrees. Line a rimmed baking sheet with parchment paper. Place the nuts, parsley, and lemon juice in a food processor and pulse until the mixture is combined and looks like crumbs. Spread mixture onto a plate.

Brush each fillet with avocado oil. Then press both sides of the fish into the nut mixture. Sprinkle with garlic, salt, and pepper. Bake for 10 to 15 minutes, until the top is crisp and slightly golden brown. Squeeze lemon over the top before serving. Serve with a side salad, cauliflower rice, or sautéed bok choy. (2 servings)

Serve with cauliflower rice (100 calories; 5 grams net carbs), sautéed bok choy (90 calories; 2 grams net carbs), a side salad made with 1 cup lettuce, ½ avocado, 1 tablespoon olive oil, 1 teaspoon vinegar, and lemon juice to taste (241 calories; 2 grams net carbs) or with lettuce, tomato, cucumbers, 1 tablespoon olive oil, and 1 teaspoon vinegar (145 calories; 4 grams net carbs).

Mediterranean-keto:

4-ounce filet only—calories: 480; net carbs: 3 grams

Strictly keto: No modifications needed.

Zoodles

2 to 3 medium zucchinis

1 tablespoon grass-fed ghee

3 tablespoons extra-virgin olive oil

1 small clove garlic, pressed

Italian herbs (optional)

Salt and pepper

Rinse the zucchini and cut off both ends. Push the zucchini through a spiral slicer (spiralizer). Heat ghee and oil in a large skillet over medium heat. Add garlic and cook for 1 minute. Add the zucchini noodles and Italian herbs. Toss to coat in the garlic butter. Cook for 1 to 5 minutes to desired doneness. Season with salt and pepper. Serve with protein of choice or as a side to any dish. (2 servings)

Mediterranean-keto:

1 cup—calories: 237; net carbs: 1 gram

Strictly keto: No modifications needed.

Red Curry Chicken

2 tablespoons avocado oil

1 pound boneless, skinless chicken thighs

1 green bell pepper, sliced

1 red bell pepper, sliced

1 cup snap peas, sliced in half

1 can (14-ounce) coconut milk

1 tablespoon fish sauce (optional)

2 tablespoons red curry paste

Salt and pepper to taste

Red pepper flakes (optional)

8–10 fresh basil leaves, sliced

Heat the oil in a large skillet over medium heat. Add the chicken. Cook for 3-4 minutes per side. Remove chicken and set aside. Add bell peppers and snap peas to pan. Cook until the peppers are tender. Remove from the pan and set aside. In the same skillet, combine the coconut milk, fish sauce, and curry paste. Stir well to combine and simmer for 4 to 5 minutes. Chop the chicken into bite-sized pieces. Add chicken, peppers, peas, and basil leaves to pan. Stir and simmer for 3 to 4 minutes. Season with salt, pepper, and chili flakes. Serve over cauliflower rice if desired (100 calories; 5 grams net carbs). (3 servings)

Mediterranean-keto:

With 6 ounces chicken—calories: 698; net carbs: 12 grams

Strictly keto: Omit snap peas. Add broccoli or mushrooms instead. Suggested serving: 4 ounces chicken for women and 6 ounces chicken for men.

With 4 ounces chicken—calories: 348; net carbs: 6 grams

With 6 ounces chicken—calories: 458; net carbs: 7 grams

SNACKS AND DESSERTS

Cauliflower Hummus

1 tablespoon grass-fed ghee

1 medium cauliflower, chopped finely

3–4 garlic cloves

2 tablespoons lemon or lime juice

6 tablespoons tahini

3 tablespoons extra-virgin olive oil or avocado oil, plus more if needed

¼ teaspoon cumin

Salt and pepper to taste

Heat ghee in a sauté pan over medium heat. Add the cauliflower and cook until tender. Add garlic and cook for 1–2 minutes stirring constantly. Remove from heat and cool. Place in a food processor or blender, add remaining ingredients, and pulse until smooth, regularly scraping down the sides. If too thick, add an extra tablespoon of olive oil or water until you reach preferred consistency. Makes roughly 2 cups. (6 servings)

Mediterranean-keto:
⅓-cup serving—calories: 194; net carbs: 6 grams

Strictly keto: No modifications needed.

Zingy Avocado Dip

2 medium avocados

1½ teaspoons lemon juice

¼ teaspoon red pepper flakes

Garlic powder, onion powder, or cumin (optional)

Fresh chopped cilantro (optional)

Salt and pepper to taste

In a food processor, blend all ingredients until smooth. Serve with sliced peppers, celery, or jicama. This dip will keep in the fridge for up to 3 days. (4 servings)

Mediterranean-keto:
½-cup serving—calories: 117; net carbs: 2 grams

Strictly keto: No modifications needed.

Nutty Granola Bars

½ cup chopped almonds

1 tablespoon chia seeds

6 tablespoons ground flaxseed meal

6 tablespoons mixed seeds (sunflower, pumpkin, sesame, etc.)

½ teaspoon stevia (debittered) or 1 tablespoon erythritol (or to taste)

¼ cup shredded coconut

Pinch salt

¼ teaspoon cinnamon (optional)

½ cup almond butter (or any nut or seed butter)

¼ cup avocado oil

Line an 8-inch square pan with parchment paper. In a medium bowl, stir together the dry ingredients. In a small microwave-safe bowl, combine the almond butter and avocado oil. Heat 30 seconds to 1 minute. Whisk well. Pour into the dry mixture and stir well. Firmly press the batter into the pan. Refrigerate until firm. Cut into 12 bars. (12 servings)

Mediterranean-keto:

1 bar—calories: 181; net carbs: 2 grams

Strictly keto: Use macadamia nuts and macadamia nut butter in place of almonds and almond butter.

Smoked Salmon and Cucumber Bites

4 ounces goat cheese

2 tablespoons extra-virgin olive oil, plus extra for drizzling

1 tablespoon minced capers

1 tablespoon minced red onion

1 teaspoon dried dill

Red pepper flakes or chili powder (optional)

6 ounces smoked wild-caught Alaskan salmon (Biltmore is my favorite brand)

Cucumber slices (about a dozen)

Salt and pepper to taste

In a small bowl, combine the goat cheese, olive oil, capers, onion, dill, and red pepper flakes. Mix well. Cut smoked salmon into 1-inch pieces. Place one piece of salmon on each cucumber slice. Add dollop of goat cheese mixture on top. Drizzle with olive oil and sprinkle with salt and pepper. (4 servings)

Mediterranean-keto:

Calories: 287; net carbs: 1 gram

Strictly keto: No modifications needed.

Keto Crackers

1 cup almond flour

3 tablespoons small seeds of your liking (sesame seeds, flaxseeds, hemp seeds, fennel seeds)

¼ teaspoon baking soda

Salt and pepper to taste

1 large egg, at room temperature

1 tablespoon extra-virgin olive oil

Preheat the oven to 350. Line a baking sheet with parchment paper. Combine dry ingredients in a large bowl. Stir well. In a small bowl, whisk the egg and olive oil. Pour into the dry ingredients. Mix well, then form a ball with the dough. Between pieces of parchment or plastic wrap, roll the dough to about ⅛-inch thick and shape into a rectangle. Cut the dough into 18 squares. Place onto baking sheet and bake for 10–15 minutes, until crispy and slightly golden. Store in an airtight container in the refrigerator for up to 4 days. Yields 18 crackers. One serving is 6 crackers.

Mediterranean-keto:

Calories: 236; net carbs: 4 grams

Strictly keto: No modifications needed.

Chocolate Peanut Butter Power Balls

¼ cup natural unsweetened peanut butter or almond butter

1 tablespoon erythritol or ½ teaspoon stevia (debittered)

2 tablespoons blanched almond flour

¼ teaspoon vanilla extract

1 teaspoon flaxseeds

¼ cup sugar-free chocolate chips (such as Lilly's)

1½ teaspoons MCT oil

Line a plate with parchment paper. Mix all ingredients except chocolate chips and oil. Scoop peanut butter mixture into 10 balls and roll them between your hands. Place them on a parchment-lined plate and put in the freezer for 30 minutes. Melt chocolate chips in a small microwave-safe bowl and mix in the MCT oil. Remove the peanut butter balls from the freezer. Dip the balls one at a time into the melted chocolate. Place balls back on parchment-lined plate. Return to freezer for 10 minutes, until the chocolate is solid. Store in freezer for up to 6 months. (10 servings)

Mediterranean-keto:

1 ball—calories: 66; net carbs: 3.2 grams

Strictly keto: Swap peanut butter for almond or mac nut butter.

1 ball—calories: 66; net carbs: 2.7 grams

Frozen Lemon Cream

½ cup lemon juice

1–2 teaspoons stevia (debittered)

4 pastured organic eggs

4 tablespoons grass-fed ghee

4 tablespoons avocado oil

2 teaspoons unflavored grass-fed powdered gelatin

Combine all the ingredients in a saucepan. Heat over low heat until just before the mixture comes to a boil, but DO NOT boil. Cool slightly. Pour into ramekins or ice cube tray and freeze. Eat like ice cream in ½ cup servings. (4 servings)

Mediterranean-keto:

Calories: 308; net carbs: 3 grams

Strictly keto: No modifications needed.

Chia Seed Pudding

1½ cups unsweetened vanilla almond, coconut, or oat milk

1 tablespoon erythritol or 1 teaspoon stevia (debittered)

¼ cup chia seeds

1 teaspoon orange zest (optional)

Blueberries, raspberries, or strawberries (optional)

Sliced almonds (optional)

Whisk milk and sweetener well in a medium bowl. Add the chia seeds and mix well. Set aside for 10–15 minutes. Stir again to break up any chia seed clumps. Add orange zest if using. Cover and refrigerate overnight. Divide between two bowls or glasses. Serve topped with berries and nuts. Also great for breakfast! (2 servings)

Mediterranean-keto:

¾-cup serving (with toppings)—calories: 253; net carbs: 6 grams

Strictly keto: Use almond milk.

Keto Molten Lava Cake

2 ounces stevia-sweetened dark chocolate (at least 70 percent cacao)

2 ounces unsalted almond butter

2 pasture-raised eggs

2 tablespoons erythritol (or to taste)

1 tablespoon super-fine almond flour

Heat oven to 350 degrees. Grease 2 ramekins with avocado oil.

Melt the chocolate and almond butter in a microwave-safe dish and stir well. In a separate bowl, beat eggs well with a mixer. Add eggs and sweetener to the chocolate mixture and mix well. Then add almond flour and stir until combined. Pour the batter into the ramekins. Bake for about 9 to 10 minutes. Let it sit 1 minute, then flip onto individual plates. Serve warm. (2 servings)

Mediterranean-keto:

1 cake—calories: 365; net carbs: 3 grams

Strictly keto: No modifications needed.

CONCLUSION

I F YOU WERE to ask me how we can live to 120 years of age, I would answer the Mediterranean-keto lifestyle. It's that good. The Mediterranean-keto lifestyle is the healthiest long-term lifestyle choice that is available today. And it's based on decades of research and millions of lives impacted for the better. For as long as God has me here on earth, that is my lifestyle health plan. That's where I will be, and I highly recommend the Mediterranean-keto lifestyle to virtually everyone.

And if you were to ask me what the best weight loss plan is, the best treatment for most sicknesses, and the best prevention of disease, I would answer the healthy keto diet. It's amazingly good and superbly effective. There is nothing better.

And you have both in your hands!

What makes this additionally incredible is the fact that you can seamlessly shift from the healthy keto diet over into the Mediterranean-keto lifestyle. It's like they were made for each other. That is why I suggest to most people that after they achieve their desired weight and other health goals with the healthy keto diet (part 1), they immediately jump over to the Mediterranean-keto lifestyle (part 2). From then on, it's a healthy lifestyle journey.

Wherever you are, whether you want to get on the healthy keto diet or move into the Mediterranean-keto lifestyle, I wish you the best. I'll see you along the way.

Appendix A

RECOMMENDED SUPPLEMENTS

T HE FOLLOWING SUPPLEMENTS are beneficial for your health and may aid in healthy weight loss.

- Divine Health oleocanthal capsules—a powerful polyphenol compound found in extra-virgin olive oil that is pressed in Greece.

- Omega-3 (fish oil): at least 1,000 milligrams per day (Aim for 2:1 ratio of EPA/DHA.)

- Fiber in the form of psyllium husk powder or Fiberzone: 1–2 tablespoons per day

- Exogenous ketones (Instant Ketones): as needed to push through keto flu or during intense exercise

- Vitamin D_3: 2,000 international units (IUs)

- Vitamin K_2: 100 micrograms per day

- A good multivitamin, such as Enhanced Multivitamin (See later in this list.)

- Methylated B complex: MTHF contains the active forms of the B vitamins, including: methylated folate, methylcobalamin, pyridoxal 5-phosphate in optimal dosages

- Magnesium: 350–400 milligrams per day (best at night, as it helps you sleep)

- Collagen protein (Keto Zone Collagen Powder, chocolate and vanilla)

Divine Health Supplements (available at shop.drcolbert.com or by calling 407-732-6952):

- Fiber Zone: great-tasting psyllium husk powder with prebiotics (inulin), available flavors: berry or unflavored (contains soluble and insoluble fibers)

- Green Supremefood: a whole food nutritional powder with fermented grasses and vegetables

- Red Supremefood: a whole food nutritional powder with antiaging fruits

- Beyond Biotic: a powerful probiotic to help restore a leaky gut; contains Bifidobacterium breve, Bifidobacterium lactis, and Lactobacillus plantarum. Available from drcolbert.com

- Ketosis strips

- Instant Ketones contains Betahydroxybuterate (BHB), a key ingredient that speeds up the process of entering ketosis and usually pulls people out of keto flu. It typically takes two to fourteen days to enter ketosis, but Instant Ketones can help you enter ketosis almost immediately. A coconut flavor hides the salty flavor that comes with BHB. Start by taking ½ scoop in water or a smoothie and gradually increase to a full scoop once or twice as needed.

- Instant ketone capsules also contain BHB; take two or three capsules as needed to help suppress appetite, to help you get back into ketosis, or to relieve keto flu.

- Keto Zone hydrolyzed collagen (vanilla and chocolate). Hydrolyzed collagen is composed of chicken collagen, containing Type I collagen and Type II collagen. As you age, your body slowly loses collagen, which is found throughout the body (hair, nails, joints, bones, heart, and skin). Your body's joints and skin repair at night, so it's best to take one scoop in any liquid twice a day or an hour before bedtime.

- Enhanced Multivitamins contain the active forms of the vitamins with chelated minerals for better absorption of the minerals.

- MCT oil powder is made of healthy fats that help support a healthy heart and brain. MCT oil also helps the liver produce ketone bodies, which put the body into ketosis and set the body up to burn fat. Take about 1 teaspoon to 2 tablespoons of MCT oil powder in coffee, or mix with any hot liquid to avoid clumping. Flavors include coconut cream, hazelnut, French vanilla, and chocolate.

- MCT oil capsules have the MCT oil in capsule form to help you keep in ketosis. I call these MCT oil capsules "keto on the go."

- Fat-Zyme is a digestive enzyme designed to break down fats and vegetables.

- Thyroid Zone, a natural supplement that supports the thyroid gland

WHAT TO DO WHEN YOUR WEIGHT LOSS PLATEAUS

L IKE STEPS, IT is natural for weight loss to hit plateaus, and then after a minor adjustment, weight loss continues. If your weight loss has stalled or plateaued for three to four weeks, then go through this checklist and adjust as needed.

Plateaus are normal when losing weight, but there are a limited number of reasons that might happen. Carefully and honestly evaluate yourself as you consider the following.

- Am I eating too many carbs? Even healthy carbs count. At the macro level, 5 percent of your daily intake coming from healthy carbs should be enough to burn fat for most anyone. That's 20 grams of healthy net carbs per day. Odds are your carb intake has crept up and is greater than 5 percent (20 grams).

- Am I consuming too much protein? If you eat an excessive amount of protein, the body will convert the excess protein to carbs, and that can throw you out of ketosis. Usually 3–4 ounces of protein per meal for women and 3–6 ounces of protein per meal for men is adequate. Some people need less.

- Am I drinking enough water? Not drinking enough water can slow weight loss down. Increase your water intake to at least six to eight glasses per day.

- Am I eating too many nuts? Eating too many nuts, which may have excessive net carbs, can knock you out of ketosis. Or maybe the excessive proteins from too many nuts are converting to sugar, which definitely would stop ketosis and weight loss.

- Do I need to start exercising? Consider adding brisk walking to your routine. Start with ten to twenty minutes of walking three times each week. You'll want to eventually increase it to thirty minutes or more five days a week, but for now this is a good start. But just walk; don't run. Also, if you are able, find a walking partner for accountability.

- Am I eating too much dairy? Dairy is often the culprit for slowing down and even stalling weight loss. Look at what you've been eating. Adjust if necessary.

- Am I eating enough fat? Double-check your 75 percent fats intake. Are you still on target? Adding more olive oil or avocado oil to meals is often the answer. For women, 75 percent of 1,600 total calories as fat is 10 tablespoons per day (3.33 tablespoons per meal). For men, 75 percent of 2,400 total calories as fat is 15 tablespoons per day (5 tablespoons per meal).

- Am I eating too much food (calories)? Maybe you are simply eating too much food. Look at your daily intake. Are you on target (1,600 calories per day for women and 2,000–2,400 calories per day for men)? Count your calories for a few days to check yourself.

- Am I consuming artificial sweeteners? Fake sugars are notorious for knocking you out of ketosis. Examine your food and drinks closely.

- Am I eating hidden sugars? Examine your food and drinks. Nut butters, for example, which are great for fat and protein intake, often have sugar added and may even have excessive carbs.

- Do I need to increase my exercise? If you want to increase your exercise (beyond the assumed twenty-minute walks at least three times a week), increase your walks to thirty minutes four or five times a week. Do more aerobic exercise, ride a bike, swim, and so on.

- Do I need to begin intermittent fasting? On a keto diet you will feel full longer and can usually skip meals, especially breakfasts. This increases your fat burning. Maintain your macros as you go. Many of my female patients are able to break through their weight loss plateaus by eating their last meals between 5:00 and 6:00 p.m.

- Am I under too much stress? Stress releases cortisol, which can cause weight gain. Stress may be unavoidable, so learn to practice techniques that calm you. Meditation, praise music, prayer, laughter, sleep, reading books, watching funny movies or TV shows, drinking tea, turning off technology, using essential oils, playing with your grandkids, or journaling are all good ways to decrease stress. If you are able to fix the situation and remove the stressor, that is always the best option. (My book *Stress Less* is a good resource if you need to break free from stress in your life.)

- Am I experiencing hormone fluctuations? Women have hormone fluctuations during their menstrual cycles, especially during their menstrual periods, and this can slow down weight loss (typically for a week). If this happens, be aware, but press on.

- Am I getting enough sleep? Getting a good night's sleep, seven to eight hours, is vital. Some people need less sleep, but odds are you need to regularly get at least seven to eight hours of sleep each night.

- Do I have a sluggish thyroid? Consult your doctor for this or read my book *Dr. Colbert's Hormone Health Zone*, but a sluggish thyroid is common (especially in women) as we age. Symptoms often include cold hands and feet, losing the outer eyebrows, a lower body temperature, constant fatigue, weight gain, and dry skin. A natural thyroid supplement is usually the answer here.

- Am I consuming too much sodium? Too much salt can slow down your weight loss. I've seen it happen. Look closely at your food intake, and you may need to cut back on the salt and salty seasonings you might be using.

- Am I exercising too much? If you do high-intensity exercise, your body has to burn glucose for energy (protein and fat burn too slowly), so you will need to increase your carbs before a workout. (Or take MCT oil powder or Instant Ketones before a workout.) Otherwise, your body will crash, you may need to sleep, and you may feel sick. All you need to do is increase your carbs before or on those high-intensity-workout days. Eventually you will find the balance. It's best to avoid high-intensity workouts until you achieve your weight loss goals, or you will probably have to increase your carbs before your workouts.

WHAT BUMPS YOU OUT OF KETOSIS?

THERE ARE ONLY a limited number of reasons your body will not be in ketosis, and they all have to do with the macronutrient breakdown for your daily food intake on your healthy keto diet. As long as your carb intake is down around 5 percent, or 20 grams a day, you should remain in ketosis.

Here are five of the most common reasons people bump themselves out of ketosis:

1. Not consuming enough fat (the goal is 75 percent)—
   This is often a lack of olive oil, but make sure you are getting the right amount of fats per meal per day. For a woman on 1,600 calories a day, that is 10 tablespoons of fat a day, or 3.33 tablespoons per meal. For men, it's about 15 tablespoons a day, or 5 tablespoons per meal.

2. Eating too much protein (the goal is 20 percent)—
   Remember, if you eat too much protein, the extra protein converts to sugar.

3. Eating too many carbs (the goal is 5 percent)—This is only 20 grams a day or equivalent to 1.5 slices of bread. It's not much, so monitor your carb intake carefully for a few days. Also, watch for those carbs that can sneak in with nut butters, artificial sweeteners, and sauces.

4. Eating too much (practice eating until satisfied)—Dial back your total food intake by 5–10 percent, or about 1,600 calories a day for women and 2,000–2,400 calories a day for men. That will adjust all your macros. Chew

each bite twenty to thirty times. Put your fork down between bites, and enjoy good conversation with family.

5. Unexpected stressors (be patient, ketosis will kick in)—This is often out of your control, but rest assured that ketosis will happen. Keep moving forward.

WHAT TO STOCK IN YOUR FRIDGE AND PANTRY

H ERE ARE SOME of the many food choices for your fridge and pantry that are ideally suited for a healthy keto diet and the Mediterranean-keto lifestyle:

- oils—olive and avocado oils especially (in dark glass containers); MCT oil (powder or liquid); cold-pressed almond, walnut, and macadamia oils; and extra-virgin coconut oil

- vegetables—avocado, arugula, cabbage, cucumbers, broccoli, celery, spinach, kale, chard, seaweed, romaine, artichokes, bean sprouts, green beans, Brussels sprouts, olives, radish, cauliflower, greens (collard, mustard, dandelion), asparagus, garlic, mushrooms, onions (of all sorts), summer squashes (yellow squash, zucchini), peppers, eggplant, and tomatoes

- low-sugar fruits—strawberries, raspberries, blackberries, blueberries, limes, lemons, plums, clementines, kiwi, cantaloupe, watermelon

- eggs (organic and/or free-range)

- fresh/dried herbs—ginger, oregano, basil, cilantro, parsley, thyme, rosemary, sage, mint, bay leaves, chili powder, cumin, curry powder, paprika, black pepper, dillweed, cayenne pepper, red pepper flakes, cinnamon, cardamom, and so on

- nuts/seeds—almonds, walnuts, Brazil nuts, peanuts, pecans, macadamias, cashews, hazelnuts, pine nuts, pistachios, chia, flax, hemp, poppy, pumpkin, safflower, sesame, sunflower, and more

- pickled/fermented foods—kefir (especially goat and sheep), dill pickles, kimchi, sauerkraut, miso, apple cider vinegar, banana peppers, capers, olives, pickled jalapeños, and more

- condiments—mustard, avocado mayo, pesto sauce, low- or no-sugar hot sauces, sugar-free ketchup, marinara sauce, low-carb Italian dressing, vanilla extract, tomato paste, red wine vinegar, balsamic vinegar, apple cider vinegar

- meats—pasture-raised poultry and eggs; wild or sustainably harvested fish, oysters, etc.; grass-fed beef, bison, pork, sheep, goat, etc.; wild deer, rabbit, elk, and so on

- dairy (to be limited to less than 10 percent of your total daily fat intake)—feta, grass-fed ghee, grass-fed butter, sour cream, heavy whipping cream, cheese, cream cheese, unsweetened yogurt, almond milk, coconut milk

- broths—chicken, beef, bone

- natural sweeteners—stevia, monk fruit, erythritol

- coffee, tea, and water (filtered)

- fiber (psyllium husk powder)

- dark chocolate (70 percent or higher cacao)

- healthy carbs to be added in the Mediterranean-keto lifestyle—beans (black, green, snap, pinto, red, kidney, garbanzo, lima, navy, white, lupini), lentils, peas (green and black-eyed), sweet potatoes, yams, cassava, taro root, gluten-free bread or gluten-free pasta, basmati white rice, millet bread, low-sugar fruits, and other healthy carbs

- supplements (See appendix A, "Recommended Supplements.")

TESTS YOU CAN ASK YOUR DOCTOR TO REQUEST

H ERE ARE SEVERAL of the levels I check and tests I request for many of my patients:

- levels of vitamin D3 using 25-hydroxy (25 OH) vitamin D test

- vitamin B_{12} levels

- the inflammatory marker hs-CRP

- the liver using a comprehensive metabolic panel

- the complete blood count (CBC)

- the lipid panel

- a cholesterol NMR lipoprofile test, an oxidized LDL cholesterol test, and a lipoprotein(a) test if cholesterol levels remain elevated

- thyroid function by testing free T3, TSH, reverse T3, and TPO antibodies

- the ferritin level (to check iron stores)

- hemoglobin A1C (which checks long-term blood sugar and insulin resistance)

- sex hormone levels for men (total and free testosterone and estradiol) and for women (FSH, estradiol, and testosterone)

Note: You don't need a blood test to start the healthy keto diet or the Mediterranean-keto lifestyle.

Note: When your weight loss stalls, this is often a good time to do thyroid tests, HbA1C tests to check for insulin resistance, and hs-CRP tests to check for chronic inflammation.

FOODS THAT CONTAIN GLUTEN AND USUALLY STOP WEIGHT LOSS

GLUTEN AND DAIRY are the most common allergens. Gluten is a protein found in certain grains and most breads, pastas, bagels, pretzels, cereals, cakes, cookies, and processed foods. Grains with gluten:

- wheat
- rye
- barley
- triticale (a hybrid of wheat and rye)

Fruits and vegetables that may include gluten:

- canned (the sauce may contain gluten)
- frozen (flavoring and sauces may contain gluten)
- dried (may have added gluten ingredients)
- pre-chopped (may be cross-contaminated with gluten)

Proteins that may or do include gluten:

- hot dogs, pepperoni, sausage, salami, bacon
- vegetarian burgers
- lunch meats/cold cuts
- ground meats

- microwavable TV dinners
- breaded meats of any kind (contain gluten)
- proteins with soy sauce (contain gluten)
- seitan (contains gluten)

Dairy that may or do include gluten:

- flavored milks and yogurts
- processed cheese products, like cheese sauces and spreads
- ice cream if additives have gluten
- malted milk drinks (contain gluten)

Fats and oils that may include gluten:

- cooking sprays
- oils with added flavors and spices

Beverages that may or do include gluten:

- drinks with added flavorings
- pre-made smoothies
- beers, ales, and lagers (these are made from grains)
- wine coolers (contain gluten)

Spices, sauces, and condiments that may or do include gluten:

- ketchup and mustard
- Worcestershire sauce
- tomato sauce
- relish and pickles

- barbecue sauce
- mayonnaise
- salad dressing
- pasta sauce
- dry spices
- salsa
- stock and bouillon cubes
- marinades
- gravy and stuffing mixes
- rice vinegar
- wheat-based soy sauce (contains gluten)
- teriyaki sauce (contains gluten)
- malt vinegar (contains gluten)[1]

A Personal Note

FROM DON COLBERT, MD

GOD DESIRES TO heal you of disease. His Word is full of promises that confirm His love for you and His desire to give you His abundant life. His desire includes more than physical health for you; He wants to make you whole in your mind and spirit as well as through a personal relationship with His Son, Jesus Christ.

If you haven't met my best friend, Jesus, I would like to take this opportunity to introduce Him to you. It is very simple. If you are ready to let Him come into your life and become your best friend, all you need to do is sincerely pray this prayer:

> *Lord Jesus, I want to know You as my Savior and Lord. I believe You are the Son of God and that You died for my sins. I also believe You were raised from the dead and now sit at the right hand of the Father praying for me. I ask You to forgive me for my sins and change my heart so that I can be Your child and live with You eternally. Thank You for Your peace. Help me to walk with You so that I can begin to know You as my best friend and my Lord. Amen.*

If you have prayed this prayer, you have just made the most important decision of your life. I rejoice with you in your decision and your new relationship with Jesus. Please contact my publisher at pray4me@charismamedia.com so that we can send you some materials that will help you become established in your relationship with the Lord. We look forward to hearing from you.

NOTES

PREFACE

1. "Prevalence of Current Tobacco Use Among Persons Aged 15 Years and Older (Age-Standardized Rate)," World Health Organization, accessed September 2, 2021, https://www.who.int/data/gho/data/indicators/indicator-details/GHO/age-standardized-prevalence-of-current-tobacco-smoking-among-persons-aged-15-years-and-older.

2. "Burden of Cigarette Use in the U.S.," Centers for Disease Control and Prevention, accessed September 22, 2021, https://www.cdc.gov/tobacco/campaign/tips/resources/data/cigarette-smoking-in-united-states.html.

3. "World Data Table," World Health Organization, accessed September 2, 2021, https://www.who.int/cardiovascular_diseases/en/cvd_atlas_29_world_data_table.pdf; "Global Cancer Data by Country," World Cancer Research Fund, 2018, https://www.wcrf.org/dietandcancer/global-cancer-data-by-country/; "Prevalence of Obesity Among Adults, BMI >= 30 (Age-Standardized Estimate) (%)," World Health Organization, accessed September 2, 2021, https://www.who.int/data/gho/data/indicators/indicator-details/GHO/prevalence-of-obesity-among-adults-bmi-=-30-(age-standardized-estimate)-(-).

INTRODUCTION

1. Rena R. Wing and Suzanne Phelan, "Long-Term Weight Loss Maintenance," *American Journal of Clinical Nutrition* 82, no. 1 (July 2005): 222S–225S, https://doi.org/10.1093/ajcn/82.1.222S.

2. Mark Hyman, *Eat Fat, Get Thin* (New York: Little, Brown and Company, 2016), 75, https://www.amazon.com/Eat-Fat-Get-Thin-Sustained/dp/0316338834?asin=0316338834&revisionId=&format=4&depth=1.

CHAPTER 1

1. "Dietary Guidelines for Americans," USDA, December 2020, https://www.dietaryguidelines.gov/sites/default/files/2021-03/Dietary_Guidelines_for_Americans-2020-2025.pdf.

2. Mark Hyman, *The Pegan Diet* (New York: Little, Brown Spark, 2021), 132, https://www.amazon.com/Pegan-Diet-Principles-Reclaiming-Nutritionally/dp/031653708X.

3. Will Cole, *Ketotarian* (New York: Avery, 2018), 21, https://www.amazon.com/Ketotarian-Mostly-Plant-Based-Cravings-Inflammation/dp/0525537171.

4. Hyman, *The Pegan Diet*, 87.

5. "Obesity Update 2017," OECD, 2017, https://www.oecd.org/els/health-systems/Obesity-Update-2017.pdf.

6. "Obesity and Overweight," Centers for Disease Control and Prevention, accessed September 3, 2021, https://www.cdc.gov/nchs/fastats/obesity-overweight.htm.

7. Cheryl D. Fryar, Margaret D. Carroll, and Cynthia L. Ogden, "Prevalence of Overweight, Obesity, and Severe Obesity Among Adults Aged 20 and Over: United States, 1960–1962 Through 2015–2016," Centers for Disease Control and Prevention, September 2018, https://www.cdc.gov/nchs/data/hestat/obesity_adult_15_16/obesity_adult_15_16.pdf.

8. "National Diabetes Statistics Report, 2020," Centers for Disease Control and Prevention, accessed September 3, 2021, https://www.cdc.gov/diabetes/data/statistics-report/index.html.

9. Cole, *Ketotarian*, 23.

10. Fanfan Zheng et al., "HbA1c, Diabetes and Cognitive Decline: The English Longitudinal Study of Ageing," *Diabetologia* 61, no. 4 (2018): 839–848, https://dx.doi.org/10.1007%2Fs00125-017-4541-7.

11. Saion Chatterjee et al., "Type 2 Diabetes as a Risk Factor for Dementia in Women Compared With Men: A Pooled Analysis of 2.3 Million People Comprising More Than 100,000 Cases of Dementia," *Diabetes Care* (December 2015): dc15–1588, https://doi.org/10.2337/dc15-1588; Weili Xu et al., "The Effect of Borderline Diabetes on the Risk of Dementia and Alzheimer's Disease," *Diabetes* 56, no. 1 (January 2007): 211–216, https://doi.org/10.2337/db06-0879.

12. Edward Giovannucci et al., "Diabetes and Cancer," *Diabetes Care* 33, no. 7 (2010): 1674–1685, https://dx.doi.org/10.2337%2Fdc10-0666; Etan Orgel and Steven D. Mittelman, "The Links Between Insulin Resistance, Diabetes, and Cancer," *Current Diabetes Reports* 13, no. 2 (2013): 213–222, https://dx.doi.org/10.1007%2Fs11892-012-0356-6; Steven S. Coughlin et al., "Diabetes Mellitus as a Predictor of Cancer Mortality in a Large Cohort of US Adults," *American Journal of Epidemiology* 159, no. 12 (June 2004): 1160–1167, https://doi.org/10.1093/aje/kwh161.

13. Hyman, *The Pegan Diet*, 131.

14. Joana Araújo, Jianwen Cai, and June Stevens, "Prevalence of Optimal Metabolic Health in American Adults: National Health and Nutrition Examination Survey 2009–2016," *Metabolic Syndrome and Related Disorders* 17, no. 1 (February 2019): 46–52, https://doi.org/10.1089/met.2018.0105.

15. Aaron Lerner and Patricia Wusterhausen, "The World Incidence and Prevalence of Autoimmune Diseases Is Increasing," *International Journal of Celiac Disease* 3, no. 4 (December 2015): 151–155, http://dx.doi.org/10.12691/ijcd-3-4-8.

16. Virginia Ladd, "Rare Autoimmune Diseases: Individually Rare, Collectively Common," AARDA, September 2019, https://www.aarda.org/rare-autoimmune-diseases-individually-rare-collectively-common/.

17. "Heart Disease," Johns Hopkins Medicine, accessed September 7, 2021, https://www.hopkinsmedicine.org/endoscopic-weight-loss-program/conditions/heart_disease.html.

18. "Lifetime Risk of Developing or Dying From Cancer," American Cancer Society, accessed September 7, 2021, https://www.cancer.org/cancer/cancer-basics/lifetime-probability-of-developing-or-dying-from-cancer.html; Cole, *Ketotarian*, 13.

19. Cole, *Ketotarian*, 21.

20. Kim Krisberg, "Heart Disease, Stroke Remain Top Killers in US, Worldwide," *The Nation's Health* 46, no. 1 (February 2016), https://www.thenationshealth.org/content/46/1/E2.

21. Sandra B. Dunbar, "Projected Costs of Informal Caregiving for Cardiovascular Disease: 2015 to 2035: A Policy Statement From the American Heart Association," *Circulation* 137, no.19 (2018): e558–e577, https://doi.org/10.1161/CIR.0000000000000570.

22. Healthline Editorial Team, "Why Heart Disease Is on the Rise in America," Healthline, updated March 10, 2017, https://www.healthline.com/health-news/why-is-heart-disease-on-the-rise.

23. Dagfinn Aune et al., "Fruit and Vegetable Intake and the Risk of Cardiovascular Disease, Total Cancer and All-Cause Mortality—a Systematic Review and Dose-Response Meta-Analysis of Prospective Studies," *International Journal of Epidemiology* 46, no. 3 (June 2017): 1029–1056, https://doi.org/10.1093/ije/dyw319.

24. Seung Hee Lee-Kwan et al., "Disparities in State-Specific Adult Fruit and Vegetable Consumption—United States, 2015," *Morbidity and Mortality Weekly Report* 66, no. 45 (November 17, 2017): 1241–1247, http://dx.doi.org/10.15585/mmwr.mm6645a1.

25. "Apples and Oranges Are the Top U.S. Fruit Choices," USDA, 2019, https://www.ers.usda.gov/data-products/chart-gallery/gallery/chart-detail/?chartId=58322.

26. "Potatoes and Tomatoes Are the Most Commonly Consumed Vegetables," USDA, 2019, https://www.ers.usda.gov/data-products/chart-gallery/gallery/chart-detail/?chartId=58340.

27. E. J. Bruno, "The Prevalence of Vitamin K Deficiency/Insufficiency, and Recommendations for Increased Intake," *Journal of Human Nutrition and Food Science* 4, no. 1 (2016): 1077, https://www.jscimedcentral.com/Nutrition/nutrition-4-1077.pdf.

28. Diane Quagliani and Patricia Felt-Gunderson, "Closing America's Fiber Intake Gap," *American Journal of Lifestyle Medicine* 11, no. 1 (January–February 2017): 80–85, https://dx.doi.org/10.1177%2F1559827615588079.

29. Hyman, *Eat Fat, Get Thin*, 96.

30. "Micronutrient Inadequacies in the US Population: An Overview," Oregon State University, accessed September 7, 2021, https://lpi.oregonstate.edu/mic/micronutrient-inadequacies/overview#potassium.

31. "Micronutrient Inadequacies in the US Population," Oregon State University.

32. "Micronutrient Inadequacies in the US Population," Oregon State University.

33. "Micronutrient Inadequacies in the US Population," Oregon State University.

34. Naveen R. Parva, "Prevalence of Vitamin D Deficiency and Associated Risk Factors in the US Population (2011–2012)," *Cureus* 10, no. 6 (June 2018): e2741, https://dx.doi.org/10.7759%2Fcureus.2741; Sunny A. Linnebur, "Prevalence of Vitamin D Insufficiency in Elderly Ambulatory Outpatients in Denver, Colorado," *American Journal of Geriatric Pharmacotherapy* 5, no. 1 (March 2007): 1–8, https://doi.org/10.1016/j.amjopharm.2007.03.005.

35. Regan L. Bailey et al., "Estimation of Total Usual Calcium and Vitamin D Intakes in the United States," *Journal of Nutrition* 140, no. 4 (April 2010): 817–822, https://doi.org/10.3945/jn.109.118539.

36. Jerrold J. Heindel and Thaddeus T. Schug, "The Obesogen Hypothesis: Current Status and Implications for Human Health," *Current Environmental Health Reports* 1 (2014): 333–340, https://doi.org/10.1007/s40572-014-0026-8.

37. Hyman, *The Pegan Diet*, 88–89.

38. Hyman, *The Pegan Diet*, 89; Matthew P. Pase et al., "Sugar- and Artificially Sweetened Beverages and the Risks of Incident Stroke and Dementia: A

Prospective Cohort Study," *Stroke* 48, no. 5 (May 2017): 1139–1146, https://doi.org/10.1161/strokeaha.116.016027.

CHAPTER 2

1. Giuseppe Passarino, Francesco De Rango, and Alberto Montesanto, "Human Longevity: Genetics or Lifestyle? It Takes Two to Tango," *Immunity and Ageing* 13 (2016): 12, https://dx.doi.org/10.1186%2Fs12979-016-0066-z.

2. Chatterjee et al., "Type 2 Diabetes as a Risk Factor for Dementia in Women Compared With Men"; Xu et al., "The Effect of Borderline Diabetes on the Risk of Dementia and Alzheimer's Disease."

3. Spencer Brooks, "The Complete Leaky Gut Diet Guide: How to Heal Your Gut," Perfect Keto, September 12, 2019, https://perfectketo.com/leaky-gut-diet/; Elise Mandl, "Does the Keto Diet Treat IBS?," Healthline, February 18, 2020, https://www.healthline.com/nutrition/keto-diet-and-ibs; Antonio Paoli et al., "Effects of a Ketogenic Diet in Overweight Women With Polycystic Ovary Syndrome," *Journal of Translational Medicine* 18 (2020): 104, https://doi.org/10.1186/s12967-020-02277-0; Marco D'Abbondanza et al., "Very Low-Carbohydrate Ketogenic Diet for the Treatment of Severe Obesity and Associated Non-Alcoholic Fatty Liver Disease: The Role of Sex Differences," *Nutrients* 12, no. 9 (2020): 2748, https://doi.org/10.3390/nu12092748; "Is Keto Diet a Good Option for GERD Patients?," Houston Heartburn & Reflux Center, accessed September 7, 2021, https://houstonheartburn.com/is-keto-diet-a-good-option-for-gerd-patients/; Rudy Mawer, "Can a Ketogenic Diet Help Fight Cancer?," Healthline, updated January 15, 2021, https://www.healthline.com/nutrition/ketogenic-diet-to-fight-cancer; Isabella D'Andrea Meira et al., "Ketogenic Diet and Epilepsy: What We Know So Far," *Frontiers in Neuroscience* 13 (2019): 5, https://dx.doi.org/10.3389%2Ffnins.2019.00005.

4. "Obesity and Overweight," Centers for Disease Control and Prevention.

5. Healthy Lifestyle Habits May Be Associated With Reduced Risk of Chronic Disease," Science Daily, August 12, 2009, https://www.sciencedaily.com/releases/2009/08/090810161906.htm.

CHAPTER 3

1. Josh Axe, *Keto Diet* (New York: Little, Brown Spark, 2019), 7, https://www.amazon.com/Keto-Diet-Balance-Hormones-Reverse/dp/0316529583.

2. Cole, *Ketotarian*, 31.

3. "Dietary Guidelines for Americans," USDA.

4. John S. O'Brien and E. Lois Sampson, "Lipid Composition of the Normal Human Brain: Gray Matter, White Matter and Myelin," *Journal of Lipid Research* 6, no. 4 (October 1965): 537–544, https://www.jlr.org/article/S0022-2275(20)39619-X/pdf.

5. Cole, *Ketotarian*, 66.

6. Ivan G. Darvey, "How Does the Ratio of ATP Yield From the Complete Oxidation of Palmitic Acid to That of Glucose Compare With the Relative Energy Contents of Fat and Carbohydrate?," *Biochemical Education* 26 (1998): 22–23, https://iubmb.onlinelibrary.wiley.com/doi/pdf/10.1016/S0307-4412(97)00046-0.

CHAPTER 4

1. Cole, *Ketotarian*, 21–22.

2. Axe, *Keto Diet*, 123.

3. Cole, *Ketotarian*, 24.

4. Hyman, *Eat Fat, Get Thin*, 161.

5. Cole, *Ketotarian*, 37.

6. Eric C. Westman et al., "The Effect of a Low-Carbohydrate, Ketogenic Diet Versus a Low-Glycemic Index Diet on Glycemic Control in Type 2 Diabetes Mellitus," *Nutrition and Metabolism* 5, no. 36 (2008), https://doi.org/10.1186/1743-7075-5-36.

7. Axe, *Keto Diet*, 116; Kris Gunnars, "Leptin and Leptin Resistance: Everything You Need to Know," Healthline, updated December 4, 2018, https://www.healthline.com/nutrition/leptin-101.

8. Andrew J. Gawron et al., "Economic Evaluations of Gastroesophageal Reflux Disease Medical Management: A Systematic Review," *Pharmacoeconomics* 32, no. 8 (August 2014): 745–758, https://dx.doi.org/10.1007%2Fs40273-014-0164-8.

9. Steven Masley, *The Mediterranean Method* (New York: Harmony Books, 2019), 79, https://www.amazon.com/Mediterranean-Method-Complete-Harness-Healthiest/dp/0593136039.

10. Masley, *The Mediterranean Method*, 98–99; Ling Xie et al., "Alzheimer's β-Amyloid Peptides Compete for Insulin Binding to the Insulin Receptor," *Journal of Neuroscience* 22 (2002): 1–5, https://www.jneurosci.org/content/jneuro/22/10/RC221.full.pdf.

11. Axe, *Keto Diet*, 9.

12. Thomas N. Seyfried, *Cancer as a Metabolic Disease* (Hoboken, NJ: John Wiley & Sons, 2012), 18, https://www.amazon.com/Cancer-Metabolic-Disease-Management-Prevention/dp/0470584920.

13. Jocelyn Tan-Shalaby, "Ketogenic Diets and Cancer: Emerging Evidence," *Federal Practitioner* 34 (February 2017): 37S–42S, https://www.ncbi.nlm.nih.gov/pmc/articles/PMC6375425/.

14. Matthew K. Taylor et al., "Feasibility and Efficacy Data From a Ketogenic Diet Intervention in Alzheimer's Disease," *Alzheimer's and Dementia* 4 (December 4, 2017): 28–36, https://dx.doi.org/10.1016%2Fj.trci.2017.11.002.

15. T. B. Vanitallie et al., "Treatment of Parkinson Disease With Diet-Induced Hyperketonemia: A Feasibility Study," *Neurology* 64, no. 4 (February 22, 2005): 728–730, https://doi.org/10.1212/01.wnl.0000152046.11390.45.

16. Eleonora Napoli, Nadia Dueñas, and Cecilia Giulivi, "Potential Therapeutic Use of the Ketogenic Diet in Autism Spectrum Disorders," *Frontiers in Pediatrics* 2 (June 30, 2014): 69, https://dx.doi.org/10.3389%2Ffped.2014.00069.

17. Axe, *Keto Diet*, 9.

18. "Nonalcoholic Fatty Liver Disease (NAFLD)," American Liver Foundation, accessed September 9, 2021, https://liverfoundation.org/for-patients/about-the-liver/diseases-of-the-liver/non-alcoholic-fatty-liver-disease/#information-for-the-newly-diagnosed.

19. Annie Guinane, "What Is the Best Diet to Treat Fatty Liver Disease?," University of Chicago Medicine, July 23, 2018, https://www.uchicagomedicine.org/forefront/gastrointestinal-articles/fatty-liver-disease-diet.

20. "Advanced Glycation End Products as Drivers of Age-Related Disease," Buck Institute, September 4, 2018, https://www.buckinstitute.org/news/advanced-glycation-end-products-as-drivers-of-age-related-disease/.

21. John C. Newman and Eric Verdin, "Ketone Bodies as Signaling Metabolite," *Cell* 25, no. 1 (January 1, 2014): 42–52, https://doi.org/10.1016/j.tem.2013.09.002.

CHAPTER 5

1. Axe, *Keto Diet*, 15.

2. "Clean Fifteen," Environmental Working Group, accessed September 9, 2021, https://www.ewg.org/foodnews/clean-fifteen.php.

3. "Dirty Dozen," Environmental Working Group, accessed September 9, 2021, https://www.ewg.org/foodnews/dirty-dozen.php.

4. Quagliani and Felt-Gunderson, "Closing America's Fiber Intake Gap."

5. Ruben Castaneda, "10 Causes of Chronic Constipation," *US News and World Report*, October 31, 2019, https://health.usnews.com/conditions/digestive-disease/constipation/articles/causes-of-chronic-constipation; "Constipation and Defecation Problems," American College of Gastroenterology, accessed September 10, 2021, https://gi.org/topics/constipation-and-defection-problems/; Thomas Sommers et al., "Emergency Department Burden of Constipation in the United States From 2006 to 2011," *American Journal of Gastroenterology* 110, no. 4 (April 2015): 572–579, https://doi.org/10.1038/ajg.2015.64.

6. Annie Stuart, "Acid Reflux Symptoms," WebMD, March 15, 2020, https://www.webmd.com/heartburn-gerd/guide/acid-reflux-symptoms#1.

7. Kathleen M. Zelman, "Fiber: How Much Do You Need?," WebMD, accessed September 10, 2021, https://www.webmd.com/diet/guide/fiber-how-much-do-you-need#1.

8. "Dietary Guidelines for Americans," USDA.

9. Mayo Clinic Staff, "Chart of High-Fiber Foods," Mayo Clinic, accessed September 10, 2021, https://www.mayoclinic.org/healthy-lifestyle/nutrition-and-healthy-eating/in-depth/high-fiber-foods/art-20050948.

10. Hyman, *Eat Fat, Get Thin*, 96.

11. Freydis Hjalmarsdottir, "12 Foods That Are Very High in Omega-3," Healthline, September 30, 2019, https://www.healthline.com/nutrition/12-omega-3-rich-foods.

12. Masley, *The Mediterranean Method*, 87.

13. Hyman, *Eat Fat, Get Thin*, 75; Glen D. Lawrence, "Dietary Fats and Health: Dietary Recommendations in the Context of Scientific Evidence," *Advances in Nutrition* 4, no. 3 (May 2013): 294–302, https://doi.org/10.3945/an.113.003657.

14. Lawrence, "Dietary Fats and Health"; M. E. Surette et al., "Evidence for Mechanisms of the Hypotriglyceridemic Effect of N-3 Polyunsaturated Fatty Acids," *Biochimica et Biophysica Acta* 1126, no. 2 (June 1992): 199–205, https://doi.org/10.1016/0005-2760(92)90291-3; Maria Luz Fernandez and Kristy L. West, "Mechanisms by Which Dietary Fatty Acids Modulate Plasma Lipids," *Journal of Nutrition* 135, no. 9 (September 2005): 2075–2078, https://doi.org/10.1093/jn/135.9.2075.

15. Tingting Shang et al., "Protective Effects of Various Ratios of DHA/EPA Supplementation on High-Fat Diet-Induced Liver Damage in Mice," *Lipids in Health and Disease* 16, no. 1 (March 29, 2017): 65, https://doi.org/10.1186/s12944-017-0461-2.

16. "Vitamin Supplements: Hype or Help for Healthy Eating," American Heart Association, accessed September 10, 2021, https://www.heart.org/en/healthy-living/healthy-eating/eat-smart/nutrition-basics/vitamin-supplements-hype-or-help-for-healthy-eating?uid=1923.

17. EFSA Panel on Dietetic Products, Nutrition and Allergies (NDA), "Scientific Opinion on the Tolerable Upper Intake Level of Eicosapentaenoic Acid (EPA), Docosahexaenoic Acid (DHA) and Docosapentaenoic Acid (DPA)," *EFSA Journal* 10, no. 7 (July 27, 2012): 2815, https://doi.org/10.2903/j.efsa.2012.2815.

CHAPTER 6

1. Cole, *Ketotarian*, 40.

2. Cole, *Ketotarian*, 41.

3. "Fat: What You Need to Know," Cleveland Clinic, accessed September 11, 2021, https://my.clevelandclinic.org/health/articles/11208-fat-what-you-need-to-know.

4. Matt Lehrer, "What Are Lipopolysaccharides (LPS)?," SelfHacked, updated January 17, 2020, https://selfhacked.com/blog/lipopolysaccharides/.

5. David Perlmutter with Kristin Loberg, *Brain Maker* (London: Yellow Kite, 2015), 56–59, https://www.amazon.com/Brain-Maker-Power-Microbes-Protect/dp/1478985550; Julie A. Gegner, Richard J. Ulevitch, and Peter S. Tobias, "Lipopolysaccharide (LPS) Signal Transduction and Clearance. Dual Roles for LPS Binding Protein and Membrane CD14," *Journal of Biological Chemistry* 270, no. 10 (March 1995): 5320–5325, https://doi.org/10.1074/jbc.270.10.5320.

6. Steven R. Gundry, *The Plant Paradox: The Hidden Dangers in "Healthy" Foods That Cause Disease and Weight Gain* (New York: HarperCollins, 2017), 64–65.

7. Richard Hagmeyer, "What Are Lipopolysaccharides, and How LPS Toxins Affect Thyroid Health?," Dr. Hagmeyer, August 25, 2014, https://www.drhagmeyer.com/what-are-lipopolysaccharides-and-how-can-they-affect-thyroid-health/.

8. Marius Trøseid et al., "Plasma Lipopolysaccharide Is Closely Associated With Glycemic Control and Abdominal Obesity," *Diabetes Care* 36, no. 11 (November 2013): 3627–3632, https://doi.org/10.2337/dc13-0451.

9. Gundry, *The Plant Paradox*, 120–125; Jeffrey M. Smith, "Survey Reports Improved Health After Avoiding Genetically Modified Foods," *International Journal of Human Nutrition and Functional Medicine* (2017), https://www.biri.org/pdf/articles/Improved-Health-After-Avoiding-GMO-Foods.pdf.

10. Awad A. Shehata et al., "The Effect of Glyphosate on Potential Pathogens and Beneficial Members of Poultry Microbiota In Vitro," *Current Microbiology* 66, no. 4 (April 2013): 350–358, https://doi.org/10.1007/s00284-012-0277-2.

11. Clémence Defois et al., "Food Chemicals Disrupt Human Gut Microbiota Activity and Impact Intestinal Homeostasis as Revealed by In Vitro Systems," *Scientific Reports* 8, no. 11006 (2018), https://doi.org/10.1038/s41598-018-29376-9.

12. Monika Kruger et al., "Glyphosate Suppresses the Antagonistic Effect of Enterococcus Spp. on Clostridium Botulinum," *Anaerobe* 20 (April 2013): 74–78, https://doi.org/10.1016/j.anaerobe.2013.01.005.

13. Elisa Zied, "Calif. to Vote on Labeling GMO Foods, but You May Already Eat Them," NBC News, November 2, 2012, https://www.nbcnews.com/health/health-news/calif-vote-labeling-gmo-foods-you-may-already-eat-them-flna1c6825713;

"Biotechnology," USDA, accessed September 12, 2021, https://www.ers.usda.gov/topics/farm-practices-management/biotechnology.

14. A. R. Vieira et al., "Foods and Beverages and Colorectal Cancer Risk: A Systematic Review and Meta-Analysis of Cohort Studies, an Update of the Evidence of the WCRF-AICR Continuous Update Project," *Annals of Oncology* 28, no. 8 (August 1, 2017): 1788–1802, https://doi.org/10.1093/annonc/mdx171; Dominika Średnicka-Tober et al., "Composition Differences Between Organic and Conventional Meat: A Systematic Literature Review and Meta-Analysis," *British Journal of Nutrition* 115, no. 6 (2016): 994–1011, https://doi.org/10.1017/S0007114515005073.

15. Ralph Loglisci, "New FDA Numbers Reveal Food Animals Consume Lion's Share of Antibiotics," Johns Hopkins Center for a Livable Future, December 23, 2010, https://livablefutureblog.com/2010/12/new-fda-numbers-reveal-food-animals-consume-lion%e2%80%99s-share-of-antibiotics.

16. Amanda J. Cross and Rashmi Sinha, "Meat-Related Mutagens/Carcinogens in the Etiology of Colorectal Cancer," *Environmental and Molecular Mutagenesis* 44, no. 1 (2004): 44–55, https://doi.org/10.1002/em.20030.

17. "Chemicals in Meat Cooked at High Temperatures and Cancer Risk," National Cancer Institute, accessed September 12, 2021, https://www.cancer.gov/about-cancer/causes-prevention/risk/diet/cooked-meats-fact-sheet.

18. A. Farhadian et al., "Effects of Marinating on the Formation of Polycyclic Aromatic Hydrocarbons (Benzo[a]pyrene, Benzo[b]fluoranthene and Fluoranthene) in Grilled Beef Meat," *Food Control* 28, no. 2 (December 2012): 420–425, https://doi.org/10.1016/j.foodcont.2012.04.034; J. S. Smith, F. Ameri, and P. Gadgil, "Effect of Marinades on the Formation of Heterocyclic Amines in Grilled Beef Steaks," *Journal of Food Science* 73, no. 6 (August 2008): 100–105, https://doi.org/10.1111/j.1750-3841.2008.00856.x.

19. Amanda S. Janesick and Bruce Blumberg, "Obesogens: An Emerging Threat to Public Health," *American Journal of Obstetrics and Gynecology* 214, no. 5 (May 2016): 559–565, https://doi.org/10.1016/j.ajog.2016.01.182.

20. Kris Gunnars, "5 Obesogens: Artificial Chemicals That Make You Fat," Healthline, updated February 6, 2018, https://www.healthline.com/nutrition/5-chemicals-that-are-making-you-fat.

21. Toru Takeuchi et al., "Positive Relationship Between Androgen and the Endocrine Disruptor, Bisphenol A, in Normal Women and Women With Ovarian Dysfunction," *Endocrine Journal* 51, no. 2 (April 2004): 165–169, https://doi.org/10.1507/endocrj.51.165; Tiange Wang et al., "Urinary Bisphenol A (BPA) Concentration Associates With Obesity and Insulin Resistance," *Journal of Clinical Endocrinology and Metabolism* 97, no. 2 (February 2012): 223–227, https://doi.org/10.1210/jc.2011-1989; Frederick S. vom Saal and Claude Hughes, "An Extensive New Literature Concerning Low-Dose Effects of Bisphenol A Shows the Need for a New Risk Assessment," *Environmental Health Perspectives* 113, no. 8 (August 2005): 926–933, https://dx.doi.org/10.1289%2Fehp.7713; Paloma Alonso-Magdalena et al., "The Estrogenic Effect of Bisphenol A Disrupts Pancreatic Beta-Cell Function In Vivo and Induces Insulin Resistance," *Environmental Health Perspectives* 114, no. 1 (January 2006): 106–112, https://doi.org/10.1289/ehp.8451; Y. Q. Huang et al., "Bisphenol A (BPA) in China: A Review of Sources,

Environmental Levels, and Potential Human Health Impacts," *Environment International* 42 (July 2012): 91–99, https://doi.org/10.1016/j.envint.2011.04.010; Caroline M. Markey et al., "Endocrine Disruptors: From Wingspread to Environmental Developmental Biology," *Journal of Steroid Biochemistry and Molecular Biology* 83, no. 1–5 (December 2002): 235–244, https://doi.org/10.1016/S0960-0760(02)00272-8.

22. Benson T. Akingbemi et al., "Phthalate-Induced Leydig Cell Hyperplasia Is Associated With Multiple Endocrine Disturbances," *Proceedings of the National Academy of Sciences of the Unites States of America* 101, no. 3 (January 2004): 775–780, https://doi.org/10.1073/pnas.0305977101.

23. Béatrice Desvergne, Jérôme N Feige, and Cristina Casals-Casas, "PPAR-Mediated Activity of Phthalates: A Link to the Obesity Epidemic?," *Molecular and Cellular Endocrinology* 304, no. 1–2 (May 25, 2009): 43–48, https://doi.org/10.1016/j.mce.2009.02.017.

24. Shanna H. Swan et al., "Decrease in Anogenital Distance Among Male Infants With Prenatal Phthalate Exposure," *Environmental Health Perspectives* 113, no. 8 (August 2005): 1056–1061, https://doi.org/10.1289/ehp.8100; Guowei Pan et al., "Decreased Serum Free Testosterone in Workers Exposed to High Levels of Di-n-butyl Phthalate (DBP) and Di-2-ethylhexyl Phthalate (DEHP): A Cross-Sectional Study in China," *Environmental Health Perspectives* 114, no. 11 (November 2006): 1643–1648, https://dx.doi.org/10.1289%2Fehp.9016; J. Toppari et al., "Environmental Effects on Hormonal Regulation of Testicular Descent," *Journal of Steroid Biochemistry and Molecular Biology* 102, no. 1–5 (December 2006): 184–186, https://doi.org/10.1016/j.jsbmb.2006.09.020; Eduardo Salazar-Martinez et al., "Anogenital Distance in Human Male and Female Newborns: A Descriptive, Cross-Sectional Study," *Environmental Health* 3, no. 1 (September 13, 2004): 8, https://doi.org/10.1186/1476-069x-3-8.

25. Qiao-Ping Wang, "Sucralose Promotes Food Intake Through NPY and a Neuronal Fasting Response," *Cell Metabolism* 24, no. 1 (July 12, 2016): 75–90, https://doi.org/10.1016/j.cmet.2016.06.010.

26. Natalie D. Luscombe-Marsh, Astrid J. P. G. Smeets, and Margriet S. Westerterp-Plantenga, "The Addition of Monosodium Glutamate and Inosine Monophosphate-5 to High-Protein Meals: Effects on Satiety, and Energy and Macronutrient Intakes," *British Journal of Nutrition* 102, no. 6 (September 2009): 929–937, https://doi.org/10.1017/s0007114509297212.

27. M. Hermanussen et al., "Obesity, Voracity, and Short Stature: The Impact of Glutamate on the Regulation of Appetite," *European Journal of Clinical Nutrition* 60 (2006): 25–31, https://doi.org/10.1038/sj.ejcn.1602263.

28. Mostafa Ibrahim et al., "Energy Expenditure and Hormone Responses in Humans After Overeating High-Fructose Corn Syrup Versus Whole-Wheat Foods," *Obesity* 26, no. 1 (January 2018): 141–149, https://doi.org/10.1002/oby.22068.

29. "How High Fructose Intake May Trigger Fatty Liver Disease," National Institutes of Health, September 15, 2020, https://www.nih.gov/news-events/nih-research-matters/how-high-fructose-intake-may-trigger-fatty-liver-disease.

30. Gunnars, "5 Obesogens."

31. "Salmon," Seafood Health Facts, accessed September 13, 2021, https://www.seafoodhealthfacts.org/seafood-choices/description-top-commercial-seafood-items/salmon.

32. Laura Reiley, "The Facts About Farmed Salmon You Wish You Didn't Know," *Tampa Bay Times*, March 21, 2018, https://www.tampabay.com/things-to-do/food/cooking/The-facts-about-farmed-salmon-you-wish-you-didn-t-know_166193900/.

33. M. Sprague, J. R. Dick, and D. R. Tocher, "Impact of Sustainable Feeds on Omega-3 Long-Chain Fatty Acid Levels in Farmed Atlantic Salmon, 2006–2015," *Scientific Reports* 6, no. 21892 (2016), https://doi.org/10.1038/srep21892.

34. "What Are PCBs?," National Ocean Service, accessed September 13, 2021, https://oceanservice.noaa.gov/facts/pcbs.html.

35. "What Are Adverse Health Effects of PCB Exposure?," Centers for Disease Control and Prevention, May 14, 2014, https://www.atsdr.cdc.gov/csem/polychlorinated-biphenyls/adverse_health.html.

36. Passarino, De Rango, and Montesanto, "Human Longevity."

37. Hyman, *The Pegan Diet*, 72.

38. Séverine Sabia et al., "Alcohol Consumption and Risk of Dementia: 23 Year Follow-Up of Whitehall II Cohort Study," *BMJ* 362 (2018): k2927, https://doi.org/10.1136/bmj.k2927; C. L. Berkowitz et al., "Clinical Application of APOE in Alzheimer's Prevention: A Precision Medicine Approach," *Journal of Prevention of Alzheimer's Disease* 5, no. 4 (2018): 245–252, https://dx.doi.org/10.14283%2Fjpad.2018.35.

39. "Alzheimer's Disease Genetics Fact Sheet," National Institute on Aging, accessed September 13, 2021, https://www.nia.nih.gov/health/alzheimers-disease-genetics-fact-sheet.

40. Jing Qian et al., "APOE-Related Risk of Mild Cognitive Impairment and Dementia for Prevention Trials: An Analysis of Four Cohorts," *PLOS Medicine* 14, no. 3 (March 2017): e1002254, https://dx.doi.org/10.1371%2Fjournal.pmed.1002254.

41. Heather Ward et al., "APOE Genotype, Lipids, and Coronary Heart Disease Risk," *Archives of Internal Medicine* 169, no. 15 (2009): 1424–1429, https://doi.org/10.1001/archinternmed.2009.234.

42. Masley, *The Mediterranean Method*, 26.

43. Hyman, *The Pegan Diet*, 94.

CHAPTER 7

1. Jacqueline D. Wright and Chia-Yih Wang, "Trends in Intake of Energy and Macronutrients in Adults From 1999–2000 Through 2007–2008," NCHS Brief, no. 49, November 2010, https://www.cdc.gov/nchs/data/databriefs/db49.pdf.

2. Oliver E. Owen and Richard W. Hanson, "Ketone Bodies," Science Direct, accessed September 13, 2021, https://www.sciencedirect.com/topics/neuroscience/ketone-bodies.

3. Cole, *Ketotarian*, 121.

4. Anahad O'Connor, "Rethinking Weight Loss and the Reasons We're 'Always Hungry,'" *New York Times*, January 7, 2016, https://well.blogs.nytimes.com/2016/01/07/rethinking-weight-loss-and-the-reasons-were-always-hungry/.

5. Amy Ramos, *The Complete Ketogenic Diet for Beginners* (Emeryville, CA: Rockridge Press, 2016), 14.

6. Ramos, *The Complete Ketogenic Diet for Beginners*, 29.

7. Axe, *Keto Diet*, 21.

8. Axe, *Keto Diet*, 21–22.

CHAPTER 8

1. Gul Ambreen, Afshan Siddiq, and Kashif Hussain, "Association of Long-Term Consumption of Repeatedly Heated Mix Vegetable Oils in Different Doses and Hepatic Toxicity Through Fat Accumulation," *Lipids in Health and Disease* 19, no. 69 (2020), https://doi.org/10.1186/s12944-020-01256-0.

2. Mayo Clinic Staff, "Trans Fat Is Double Trouble for Your Heart Health," Mayo Clinic, accessed September 13, 2021, https://www.mayoclinic.org/diseases-conditions/high-blood-cholesterol/in-depth/trans-fat/art-20046114.

3. Ramón Estruch et al., "Primary Prevention of Cardiovascular Disease With a Mediterranean Diet Supplemented With Extra-Virgin Olive Oil or Nuts," *New England Journal of Medicine* 378, no. 25 (June 21, 2018): e34, https://doi.org/10.1056/nejmoa1800389.

4. Hyman, *The Pegan Diet*, 73.

5. Michel de Lorgeril et al., "Mediterranean Diet, Traditional Risk Factors, and the Rate of Cardiovascular Complications After Myocardial Infarction," *Circulation* 99, no. 6 (1999): 779–785, https://doi.org/10.1161/01.CIR.99.6.779; "Statin Medications & Heart Disease," Cleveland Clinic, accessed September 13, 2021, https://my.clevelandclinic.org/health/articles/17506-statin-medications--heart-disease.

6. Marta Guasch-Ferré et al., "Olive Oil Intake and Risk of Cardiovascular Disease and Mortality in the PREDIMED Study," *BMC Medicine* 12, no. 78 (2014), https://doi.org/10.1186/1741-7015-12-78.

7. "Fats," American Diabetes Association, accessed September 13, 2021, https://www.diabetes.org/healthy-living/recipes-nutrition/eating-well/fats.

8. Mayo Clinic Staff, "Trans Fat Is Double Trouble for Your Heart Health"; Vandana Dhaka et al., "Trans Fats—Sources, Health Risks and Alternative Approach—a Review," *Journal of Food Science Technology* 48, no. 5 (October 2011): 534–541, https://dx.doi.org/10.1007%2Fs13197-010-0225-8.

9. E. Patterson et al., "Health Implications of High Dietary Omega-6 Polyunsaturated Fatty Acids," *Journal of Nutrition and Metabolism* 2012, no. 539426 (2012), https://doi.org/10.1155/2012/539426.

10. M. J. Reed et al., "Free Fatty Acids: A Possible Regulator of the Available Oestradiol Fractions in Plasma," *Journal of Steroid Biochemistry* 24, no. 2 (February 1986): 657–659, https://doi.org/10.1016/0022-4731(86)90134-2; Karma L. Pearce and Kelton Tremellen, "The Effect of Macronutrients on Reproductive Hormones in Overweight and Obese Men: A Pilot Study," *Nutrients* 11, no. 12 (2019): 3059, https://doi.org/10.3390/nu11123059; P. C. Calder, "Polyunsaturated Fatty Acids, Inflammation, and Immunity," *Lipids* 36, no. 9 (September 2001): 1007–1024, https://doi.org/10.1007/s11745-001-0812-7; Urszula Radzikowska et al., "The Influence of Dietary Fatty Acids on Immune Responses," *Nutrients* 11, no. 12 (December 2019): 2990, https://dx.doi.org/10.3390%2Fnu11122990; Anamaria Balić et al., "Omega-3 Versus Omega-6 Polyunsaturated Fatty Acids in the Prevention and Treatment of Inflammatory Skin Diseases," *International*

Journal of Molecular Sciences 21, no. 3 (February 2020): 741, https://dx.doi.
org/10.3390%2Fijms21030741.

11. Maria Azrad, Chelsea Turgeon, and Wendy Demark-Wahnefried, "Current Evidence Linking Polyunsaturated Fatty Acids With Cancer Risk and Progression," *Frontiers in Oncology* 3 (2013): 224, https://dx.doi.org/10.3389%2Ffonc.2013.00224.

12. Hyman, *The Pegan Diet*, 60.

13. Foundation staff, "Healthiest Cooking Oil Comparison Chart With Smoke Points and Omega 3 Fatty Acid Ratios," Baseline of Health Foundation, April 17, 2019, https://www.jonbarron.org/diet-and-nutrition/healthiest-cooking-oil-chart-smoke-points.

14. Cole, *Ketotarian*, 72.

CHAPTER 9

1. Hyman, *The Pegan Diet*, 63.
2. Hyman, *The Pegan Diet*, 64.
3. H. D. Karsten et al., "Vitamins A, E and Fatty Acid Composition of the Eggs of Caged Hens and Pastured Hens," *Renewable Agriculture and Food Systems* 25, no. 1 (2010): 45–54, https://doi.org/10.1017/S1742170509990214.
4. Suzanne Ryan, *Simply Keto* (Las Vegas, NV: Victory Belt, 2017), 53, https://www.amazon.com/Simply-Keto-Practical-Approach-Low-Carb/dp/1628602635.
5. "Grass-Fed Beef: Is It Good for You?," WebMD, accessed September 14, 2021, https://www.webmd.com/diet/grass-fed-beef-good-for-you#1.
6. Ryan, *Simply Keto*, 53.
7. Martha Clare Morris et al., "Consumption of Fish and N-3 Fatty Acids and Risk of Incident Alzheimer Disease," *Archives of Neurology* 60, no. 7 (July 2003): 940–946, https://doi.org/10.1001/archneur.60.7.940.
8. Hyman, *The Pegan Diet*, 65–66.
9. Hyman, *The Pegan Diet*, 42.
10. Hyman, *The Pegan Diet*, 45.
11. Hyman, *The Pegan Diet*, 46.
12. Hyman, *The Pegan Diet*, 21.
13. Hyman, *The Pegan Diet*, 46.
14. Piet A. van den Brandt and Leo J. Schouten, "Relationship of Tree Nut, Peanut and Peanut Butter Intake With Total and Cause-Specific Mortality: A Cohort Study and Meta-Analysis," *International Journal of Epidemiology* 44, no. 3 (2015): 1038–1049, https://doi.org/10.1093/ije/dyv039; Joan Sabaté, Keiji Oda, and Emilio Ros, "Nut Consumption and Blood Lipid Levels: A Pooled Analysis of 25 Intervention Trials," *Archives of Internal Medicine* 170, no. 9 (May 10, 2010): 821–827, https://doi.org/10.1001/archinternmed.2010.79; Luc Djoussé, Tamara Rudich, and J. Michael Gaziano, "Nut Consumption and Risk of Hypertension in US Male Physicians," *Clinical Nutrition* 28, no. 1 (February 2009): 10–14, https://dx.doi.org/10.1016%2Fj.clnu.2008.08.005.
15. Ruairi Robertson, "The Top 9 Nuts to Eat for Better Health," Healthline, September 26, 2018, https://www.healthline.com/nutrition/9-healthy-nuts.
16. "Selenium," National Institutes of Health, accessed September 14, 2021, https://ods.od.nih.gov/factsheets/Selenium-Consumer/.

17. Cole, *Ketotarian*, 74.

CHAPTER 10

1. Ramos, *The Complete Ketogenic Diet for Beginners*, 16–17.
2. Hyman, *The Pegan Diet*, 48; Gundry, *The Plant Paradox*, 43.
3. Cole, *Ketotarian*, 80.

CHAPTER 11

1. Cole, *Ketotarian*, 22–23.
2. Jeff S. Volek and Stephen D. Phinney, *The Art and Science of Low Carbohydrate Performance* (Lexington, KY: Beyond Obesity, 2012), 7.

CHAPTER 12

1. Ryan, *Simply Keto*, 39; Cole, *Ketotarian*, 126; Tyler Cartwright, "What Causes Keto Flu? (and 6 Keto Flu Remedies)," Drink LMNT, accessed September 13, 2021, https://drinklmnt.com/blogs/health/what-causes-keto-flu-and-6-keto-flu-remedies.
2. James J. DiNicolantonio, James H. O'Keefe, and William Wilson, "Subclinical Magnesium Deficiency: A Principal Driver of Cardiovascular Disease and a Public Health Crisis," *Open Heart* 5, no. 1 (2018): e000668, https://dx.doi.org/10.1136%2Fopenhrt-2017-000668.
3. Ramos, *The Complete Ketogenic Diet for Beginners*, 21.
4. Quagliani and Felt-Gunderson, "Closing America's Fiber Intake Gap."
5. Castaneda, "10 Causes of Chronic Constipation."
6. Stuart, "Acid Reflux Symptoms."
7. Ryan, *Simply Keto*, 43.
8. Belinda Lennerz and Jochen K. Lennerz, "Food Addiction, High-Glycemic-Index Carbohydrates, and Obesity," *Clinical Chemistry* 64, no. 1 (January 2018): 64–71, https://doi.org/10.1373/clinchem.2017.273532.
9. Axe, *Keto Diet*, 81.
10. Axe, *Keto Diet*, 54.

CHAPTER 14

1. Araújo, Cai, and Stevens, "Prevalence of Optimal Metabolic Health in American Adults."

CHAPTER 15

1. Lorgeril et al., "Mediterranean Diet, Traditional Risk Factors, and the Rate of Cardiovascular Complications After Myocardial Infarction"; "Statin Medications & Heart Disease," Cleveland Clinic.
2. Limor Goren et al., "(-)-Oleocanthal and (-)-Oleocanthal-Rich Olive Oils Induce Lysosomal Membrane Permeabilization in Cancer Cells," *Plos One* (August 14, 2019), https://doi.org/10.1371/journal.pone.0216024.
3. Keith Rowe, "Polyphenols: What They Are and Why You Need to Be Eating Them," BrainMD, May 7, 2020, https://brainmd.com/blog/what-are-polyphenols/; Michael Joseph, "The Top 100 Foods High in Polyphenols," Nutrition Advance, December 20, 2019, https://www.nutritionadvance.com/nutrition/top-food-sources-polyphenols/.

4. Goren et al., "(-)-Oleocanthal and (-)-Oleocanthal-Rich Olive Oils Induce Lysosomal Membrane Permeabilization in Cancer Cells."

5. Goren et al., "(-)-Oleocanthal and (-)-Oleocanthal-Rich Olive Oils Induce Lysosomal Membrane Permeabilization in Cancer Cells"; Yazan S. Batarseh and Amal Kaddoumi, "Oleocanthal-Rich Extra-Virgin Olive Oil Enhances Donepezil Effect by Reducing Amyloid-β Load and Related Toxicity in a Mouse Model of Alzheimer's Disease," *Journal of Nutritional Biochemistry* 55 (May 2018): 113–123, https://doi.org/10.1016/j.jnutbio.2017.12.006.

6. Antonio Segura-Carretero and Jose Antonio Curiel, "Current Disease-Targets for Oleocanthal as Promising Natural Therapeutic Agent," *International Journal of Molecular Sciences* 19, no. 10 (October 2018): 2899, https://dx.doi.org/10.3390%2Fijms19102899/.

7. Hyman, *The Pegan Diet*, 93.

8. "Country Trends," Seven Countries Study, accessed September 14, 2021, https://www.sevencountriesstudy.com/about-the-study/countries/country-trends/.

9. Dan Buettner, "The Island Where People Forget to Die," *New York Times*, October 28, 2012, https://www.nytimes.com/2012/10/28/magazine/the-island-where-people-forget-to-die.html.

CHAPTER 16

1. Jean A. Welsh, Saul Karpen, and Miriam B. Vos, "Increasing Prevalence of Nonalcoholic Fatty Liver Disease Among United States Adolescents, 1988–1994 to 2007–2010," *Journal of Pediatrics* 162, no. 3 (March 2013): 496–500, https://doi.org/10.1016/j.jpeds.2012.08.043.

2. M. de Lorgeril et al., "Mediterranean Diet, Traditional Risk Factors, and the Rate of Cardiovascular Complications After Myocardial Infarction: Final Report of the Lyon Diet Heart Study," *Circulation* 99, no. 6 (February 16, 1999): 779–85, https://pubmed.ncbi.nlm.nih.gov/9989963/.

3. Ramón Estruch, MD, PhD, et al., "Primary Prevention of Cardiovascular Disease With a Mediterranean Diet," *New England Journal of Medicine* 368 (2013): 1279–90, https://www.nejm.org/doi/full/10.1056/nejmoa1200303.

4. Federica Turati et al., "Glycemic Load and Coronary Heart Disease in a Mediterranean Population: The EPIC Greek Cohort Study," *Nutrition, Metabolism and Cardiovascular Diseases* 25, no. 3 (March 2015): 336–42, https://pubmed.ncbi.nlm.nih.gov/25638596/.

5. Tommaso Ballarini et al., "Mediterranean Diet, Alzheimer Disease Biomarkers, and Brain Atrophy in Old Age," *Neurology* 96, no. 24 (June 15, 2021), https://n.neurology.org/content/96/24/e2920.abstract.

6. Valentina Berti et al., "Mediterranean Diet and 3-Year Alzheimer Brain Biomarker Changes in Middle-Aged Adults," *Neurology* 90, no. 20 (May 15, 2018), https://n.neurology.org/content/90/20/e1789.

7. Cecilia Samieri et al., "The Relation of Midlife Diet to Healthy Aging: a Cohort Study," *Annals of Internal Medicine* 159, no. 9 (November 5, 2013): 584–91, https://www.ncbi.nlm.nih.gov/pmc/articles/PMC4193807/.

8. Marta Crous-Bou et al., "Mediterranean Diet and Telomere Length in Nurses' Health Study: Population Based Cohort Study," *The BMJ* 349 (December 2, 2014), https://www.bmj.com/content/349/bmj.g6674.

9. Regina Wierzejska, "Can Coffee Consumption Lower the Risk of Alzheimer's Disease and Parkinson's Disease? A Literature Review," *Archives of Medical Science* 13, no. 3 (April 1, 2017): 507–514, https://dx.doi.org/10.5114%2Faoms.2016.63599; Laura M. Stevens et al., "Association Between Coffee Intake and Incident Heart Failure Risk," *Circulation: Heart Failure* 14, no. 2 (2021): e006799, https://doi.org/10.1161/CIRCHEARTFAILURE.119.006799.

10. "U.S. News Reveals Best Diet Rankings for 2021," *U.S. News and World Report*, January 4, 2021, https://www.usnews.com/info/blogs/press-room/articles/2021-01-04/us-news-reveals-best-diet-rankings-for-2021.

CHAPTER 17

1. Masley, *The Mediterranean Method*, 78.

2. Masley, *The Mediterranean Method*, 77–78.

3. Michel de Lorgeril et al., "Mediterranean Dietary Pattern in a Randomized Trial," *Archives of Internal Medicine* 158, no. 11 (1998): 1181–1187, https://doi.org/10.1001/archinte.158.11.1181.

4. Theodora Psaltopoulou et al., "Olive Oil Intake Is Inversely Related to Cancer Prevalence: A Systematic Review and a Meta-Analysis of 13800 Patients and 23340 Controls in 19 Observational Studies," *Lipids in Health and Disease* 10, no. 127 (2011), https://doi.org/10.1186/1476-511X-10-127.

5. Estefanía Toledo et al., "Mediterranean Diet and Invasive Breast Cancer Risk Among Women at High Cardiovascular Risk in the PREDIMED Trial," *JAMA Internal Medicine* 175, no. 11 (2015): 1752–1760, https://doi.org/10.1001/jamainternmed.2015.4838.

6. Masley, *The Mediterranean Method*, 25.

7. Hyman, *Eat Fat, Get Thin*, 216.

8. Gundry, *The Plant Paradox*, 14–15.

9. Klaas Vandepoele and Yves Van de Peer, "Exploring the Plant Transcriptome Through Phylogenetic Profiling," *Plant Physiology* 137 (January 2005): 31–42, http://bioinformatics.psb.ugent.be/pdf/klpoepph.pdf.

10. "13 Surprising Health Benefits of Apples That'll Have You Eating One (or More) a Day," Best Health, September 2, 2021, https://www.besthealthmag.ca/article/health-benefits-apples/.

CHAPTER 19

1. Masley, *The Mediterranean Method*, 85.

APPENDIX F

1. Brianna Elliott, "54 Foods You Can Eat on a Gluten-Free Diet," Healthline, December 22, 2019, https://www.healthline.com/nutrition/gluten-free-foods.

INDEX

MY FREE GIFT TO YOU

Thank you for reading my book. I hope *Beyond Keto* has given you the tools you need to conquer disease and lose weight for good. Write a review, and help spread the word to others about how they also can overcome unhealthy habits forever.

As my way of saying thank you...

I am offering you the *Dr. Colbert's Healthy Gut Zone* e-book for FREE!

To get this free gift, please go to DrColbertBooks.com/freegifts.

Thank you, and God bless,

Dr. Don Colbert

SILOAM